Cognitive-Behavioral Therapy
for Anger and Aggression
in Children

Denis G.

Lawrenc

THE GUILFORD PRESS
New York   London

© 2012 The Guilford Press
A Division of Guilford Publications, Inc.
72 Spring Street, New York, NY 10012
www.guilford.com

Printed in the United States of America

This book is printed on acid-free paper.

Last digit is print number: 9 8 7 6 5 4 3 2 1

The authors have checked with sources believed to be reliable in their efforts to provide information that is complete and generally in accord with the standards of practice that are accepted at the time of publication. However, in view of the possibility of human error or changes in behavioral, mental health, or medical sciences, neither the authors, nor the editors and publisher, nor any other party who has been involved in the preparation or publication of this work warrants that the information contained herein is in every respect accurate or complete, and they are not responsible for any errors or omissions or the results obtained from the use of such information. Readers are encouraged to confirm the information contained in this book with other sources.

Library of Congress Cataloging-in-Publication Data
Sukhodolsky, Denis G.
  Cognitive-behavioral therapy for anger and aggression in children / Denis G. Sukhodolsky, Lawrence Scahill.
    p. cm.
  Includes bibliographical references and index.
  ISBN 978-1-4625-0632-3 (pbk.)
  1. Anger in children—Treatment. 2. Aggressiveness in children—Treatment. 3. Cognitive therapy for children. I. Scahill, Lawrence. II. Title.
  RJ506.A35S85 2012
  618.92′891425—dc23
                                                    2012006289

Illustrations by Deborah K. Reich

social workers, psychiatric nurse practitioners, and other professionals who provide mental health services to children. The CBT approach described in this book can be used in outpatient mental health settings, inpatient services, schools, juvenile justice programs, and other facilities where children with disruptive behavior may receive psychotherapy or counseling.

ACKNOWLEDGMENTS

This treatment has evolved from nearly two decades of clinical work and research on behavioral interventions for children with neuropsychiatric disorders complicated by disruptive behavior.

We are grateful to many colleagues without whom this book would not have been possible. The research and mentorship of Howard Kassinove, Professor and Director of the Institute for the Study and Treatment of Anger and Aggression at Hofstra University, have played a critical role in shaping our thinking about anger and its treatment. Mitchell Schare, Joseph Scardapane, Robert Motta, Bernard Gorman, and Sergei Tsytsarev of Hofstra University contributed to the initial stages of treatment development and evaluation through pilot studies and meta-analytic reviews. Ross Solomon, Sammy Richman, Igor Davidson, Arthur Golub, and Jeff Kassinove collaborated in the early studies and clinical applications of this treatment in public schools, university clinics, and inpatient units. We are also grateful to John Lochman at the University of Alabama and Eva Feindler at Long Island University, whose pioneering research on anger-control training for children and adolescents provided the foundation for our work.

The Yale Child Study Center has been fertile ground for developing and testing this treatment approach in children with neurodevelopmental disorders. We are grateful to James Leckman, Robert King, Paul Lombroso, Lawrence Vitulano, Heidi Grantz, Lily Katsovich, and Virginia Eicher for their help in implementing and evaluating this treatment in children and adolescents with Tourette syndrome. While serving as the Director of the Yale Child Study Center, Alan Kazdin offered valuable advice on refining the problem-solving component of this CBT program. Roumen Nikolov, Vladislav Ruchkin, and Elena Grigorenko collaborated on the application of CBT in the juvenile justice system. Andres Martin and Laurie Cardona encouraged the implementation of anger-control training at the Yale Children's Psychiatric Inpatient Unit. We are grateful to Joseph Woolston and Christine Dauser for discussions about the application of this treatment in the outpatient clinic. More recently, we have been piloting this treatment in children with high-functioning autism spectrum disorders complicated by noncompliance and irritability. These efforts have been supported by Fred Volkmar, Kevin Pelphrey, James McPartland, Kathy Koenig, Michael Crowley, and Linda Mayes. We would also like to thank Julie Wolf and Pamela Ventola for clinical evaluations of study participants; Joseph McGuire, Allison Gavaletz, Christopher Bailey, and Avery Voos for study coordination; and Jia Wu and Danielle Bolling for data analysis. We also acknowledge with appreciation the support of our research provided by the National Institute of Mental Health and the Tourette Syndrome Association. At The Guilford Press, Kitty Moore, Alice Broussard, and Laura Specht Patchkofsky provided editorial direction and constructive reviews that have greatly improved the content and organization of this book. Finally, we would like to acknowledge the love and support of our families: Denis's wife, Miyun, and their children, Alexander and Andrew; and Larry's wife, Sally, and their children, Katherine and Sylvia. Denis would like to give special thanks to his parents, Larisa and Gennadi, who instilled a passion for psychology and research in their son.

Contents

PARENT SESSIONS

Introduction

The word *anger* is often used as an umbrella term for various child and adolescent[1] disruptive behaviors, including explosive outbursts, quarrelling, physical aggression, and noncompliance. Some of these behaviors are common and can be developmentally appropriate, such as occasional tantrums in preschoolers or rough-and-tumble play with siblings (Jarvis, 2006). Frequent, persistent, or serious forms of disruptive behavior, however, may cause considerable social and clinical problems in children. For example, when asked about their experiences with violence, 36% of adolescents reported being in a physical fight during the past 12 months and 3.6% also reported that they were injured and had to be treated by a doctor or nurse (Eaton et al., 2006). Disruptive behavior is among the most frequent reasons for outpatient mental health referrals (Armbruster, Sukhodolsky, & Michalsen, 2004), and physical aggression is a frequent reason for psychiatric hospitalization (Rice, Woolston, Stewart, Kerker, & Horwitz, 2002). Furthermore, virtually any childhood psychiatric condition may be associated with excessive anger, irritability, and disruptive behavior.

TYPES OF DISRUPTIVE BEHAVIOR

Disruptive behaviors in children and adolescents may take various forms, but the most frequent problems include excessive (1) anger, (2) physical aggression, and (3) noncompliance. It is helpful to distinguish among these three types of disruptive behavior even though the terminology used to describe these behaviors is often used interchangeably both in lay language and the scientific literature.

---

[1] We use "children" to refer to both children and adolescents unless there is developmental distinction.

1

Anger

Anger is a negative affective state that may include altered physiological arousal and thoughts about harm or blame (Berkowitz, 1990). Anger is one of the basic emotions; healthy adults report that they get angry about once or twice per week and that their anger experiences last about 30 minutes on average (Averill, 1983; Kassinove, Sukhodolsky, Tsytsarev, & Solovyova, 1997). Anger can also vary in intensity from mild annoyance to rage and fury. Factor-analytic studies distinguish between the anger experience—that is, the inner feeling—and anger expression—that is, an individual's tendency to act on anger by showing it outwardly, suppressing it, or actively coping with it (Spielberger, 1988). On the one hand, the phenomenology of anger expression is often characterized in terms of physical and verbal aggression. For example, an angry person may express his anger by raising his voice and using profanities. On the other hand, studies with healthy adults show that talking and solving the problem are the most common behaviors associated with anger (Kassinove et al., 1997). In other words, when angry, most adults don't yell and argue, contrary to popular belief, but calmly discuss and solve the problem that made them angry.

Many brilliant minds—Aristotle, Darwin, and Freud, to name just a few—have commented on the nature of anger and its place in human psychology. However, it is only during the past two decades that considerable advances have been made in experimental anger research. This research has expanded our understanding of the phenomenology of anger and provided tools for its assessment and treatment. Several important findings in the field of anger research have been consistently replicated. For example, the facial expressions of anger are universally recognized (Ekman, 1993), and excessive and chronic anger has been found to be a risk factor in cardiovascular disease (Suls & Bunde, 2005). However, an agreed-upon definition of anger remains elusive; it has been referred to as a social role, a perception of blameworthiness, and a blueprint for aggression. In a narrow sense, the word *anger* refers to a transient emotional state that varies in intensity (from mild annoyance to fury) and duration (from a few moments to several hours) (Kassinove & Sukhodolsky, 1995).

From the developmental standpoint, various aspects of anger experience and expression emerge at different times and follow different developmental trajectories. For example, facial expressions of anger can be recognized in infants as early as 2 months old. The development of self-awareness and language, however, are prerequisites for the experience of anger and communication about this emotion to others. By the age of 2½ years most children have a variety of verbal resources including anger to communicate their emotional experiences. Temper tantrums are common in children between the ages of 18 months and 4 years and may include behaviors such as crying, stamping of feet, pushing, hitting, and kicking. In a survey of 349 families with 1- to 4-year-olds, the average frequency of tantrums ranged from five to nine per week and the average duration of a tantrum was 5 to 10 minutes (Potegal & Davidson, 2003; Potegal, Kosorok, & Davidson, 2003). The intensity and duration of tantrums tend to decrease with age, although healthy children continue to display anger and frustration through behaviors that parents often label as tantrums. This decrease in frequency of temper tantrums with age is paralleled by the development of emotion regulation skills and the acquisition of socially appropriate expressions of anger (Blanchard-Fields & Coats, 2008).

Intense and out-of-control anger outbursts may be of clinical concern in younger children (i.e., preschoolers) (Wakschlag, Tolan, & Leventhal, 2010). Extended explosive anger outbursts, which occur more often than once a week and in response to trivial provocations, may require treatment in school-age children and adolescents. Depending on the frequency and level of emotional intensity and "explosiveness" of such anger outbursts, they have been referred to as "rages" or "rage attacks" in children with severe mood dysregulation (Carlson, 2007).

Explosive outbursts and persistent irritability may also be present in children with various psychiatric conditions including disruptive behavior disorders, mood disorders, autism spectrum disorders, and tic disorders. An area of current controversy in child mental health is whether children with pervasive irritability and explosive behavior meet criteria for a bipolar spectrum disorder (Wozniak et al., 1995). On the other side of the debate, some argue that bipolar disorders are essentially episodic in nature and that chronic irritability is due to impaired ability to regulate emotion (Leibenluft, Blair, Charney, & Pine, 2003). Although this controversy remains unresolved, there has been a steady increase in the number of diagnosed cases of bipolar disorder over the past decade (Pavuluri, Birmaher, & Naylor, 2005). In response to this discussion, there is now a proposal for a new diagnostic category "Temper Dysregulation Disorder with Dysphoria" for the fifth edition of the *Diagnostic and Statistical Manual of Mental Disorders* (DSM-5), which is scheduled for publication in 2013. The proposed disorder is characterized by severe recurrent temper outbursts in response to common stressors.

Education about anger and its associated thoughts and behaviors is an important part of the cognitive-behavioral therapy (CBT) program presented in this book. The first two sessions of the manual make use of the "anger episode" model that breaks the occurrence of any anger experience into six components: triggers, thoughts, feelings, rules, actions, and outcomes. This model stems from the social-constructivist approach to anger, and it has been helpful in integrating various techniques aimed at reducing unpleasant anger and preventing disruptive behavior. For children who are not inclined to discuss their feelings at length, a simplified A-B-C approach (antecedent–behavior–consequence) can be used to teach about the triggers and consequences of excessive anger expression.

Physical Aggression

In contrast to the narrow view of anger as an emotion, and consequently an internal phenomenon, aggression is overt behavior that can result in harm to self or others. Several subtypes of aggression (e.g., impulsive, reactive, hostile, affective) have been described based on the presence of angry affect and contrasted with instrumental, proactive, or planned types of aggression that are not "fueled" by anger (Vitiello &

Stoff, 1997). Another well-known classification distinguishes between overtly confrontational antisocial behavior such as arguing and fighting and covert antisocial behaviors such as lying, stealing, and breaking rules (Achenbach, Conners, Quay, Verhulst, & Howell, 1989; Frick et al., 1993). Physical aggression was found to be a significant risk factor for early age of onset of conduct disorder (Lahey et al., 1998), later violence (Lipsey & Wilson, 1998), and other mental health problems such as attention-deficit/hyperactivity disorder (ADHD) and anxiety (Loeber, Green, Kalb, Lahey, & Loeber, 2000). Compared to physical aggression, nonaggressive antisocial behavior was shown to follow a different developmental trajectory (Maughan, Rowe, Pickles, Costello, & Angold, 2000; Nagin & Tremblay, 1999) and to predict later nonviolent criminal offenses (Kjelsberg, 2002).

In the treatment program presented in this book, children are taught how to anticipate and prevent situations that may trigger aggressive behaviors through problem solving. The treatment techniques presented in this book have been effective in reducing childhood aggressive behaviors such as pushing, punching, or kicking, which are unlikely to result in serious injury. Although these behaviors are troublesome in their own right and are among the most common reasons why children may be referred for mental health treatments, they should be distinguished from serious acts of violence and juvenile criminal behavior. A risk analysis should be conducted whenever a child presents a risk of violence to self or others. Areas for assessment include stated intent, past history of violent actions, nature of current threat, access to weapons, and effectiveness of current supervision (Borum, 2000; Borum, Fein, Vossekuil, & Berglund, 1999). Clinicians are well advised to pay special attention to the informed consent issues during these evaluations and to document all steps taken to evaluate the issue and provide appropriate treatment (Ash & Nurcombe, 2007).

Noncompliance

"Noncompliant behavior" in children is defined as a refusal to follow instructions, established rules, and quarreling with adults in the context of day-to-day activities (McMahon & Forehand, 2003). Although noncompliance is commonly reported by parents and teachers of children in the general population, it is more prevalent in clinically referred children, especially those with disruptive behavior disorders and developmental disabilities (Benson & Aman, 1999; Keenan & Wakschlag, 2004). Noncompliance is the essential feature of oppositional defiant disorder, a pattern of defiant, disobedient, and hostile behavior toward authority figures. Common examples of noncompliance include refusal to carry out expected behaviors such as chores or homework, and refusal to discontinue preferred behaviors such as watching TV or playing video games. Ignoring parental requests (often described as "not listening"), arguing, whining, and refusing to take no for an answer are common complaints in clinical practice. Although noncompliance and aggression frequently co-occur, they represent different types of disruptive behaviors that may present separate treatment targets (Sukhodolsky, Cardona, & Martin, 2005).

This treatment manual covers effective listening and communication skills in order to help a child reduce noncompliance with parental requests and find new ways to avoid or resolve conflicts with adults at school and in the community.

A NOTE ON GENDER

There are gender differences in the development of anger and aggression. For example, school-age boys are more likely than girls to engage in physical aggression and to be labeled as "angry" by teachers or parents. The prevalence rates of disruptive behavior disorders are also higher in boys. For example, in a population study of 9- to 16-year-old children, the prevalence of oppositional defiant disorder was 3.1% in boys and 2.1% in girls; the prevalence of conduct disorder was 4.2% and 1.2% for boys and girls, respectively (Costello, Mustillo, Erkanli, Keeler, & Angold, 2003). There is some evidence that developmental trajectories of conduct problems vary by gender. The average age of onset of conduct problems is later in girls compared to boys, and some studies suggest that later onset is associated with more favorable outcomes (Fergusson & Horwood, 2002). Despite a later age of onset, however, girls with conduct disorder may exhibit poor outcomes that are similar to boys who engage in antisocial behavior at a younger age (Silverthorn & Frick, 1999). Although there is increasing interest in the delinquent behavior of girls in the juvenile justice system (Office of Juvenile Justice and Delinquency Prevention, 2008), only the Oregon Multidimensional Treatment Foster Care Model was directly studied with girls with serious antisocial behavior problems (Leve, Chamberlain, & Reid, 2005). Clinical studies with large samples are needed to examine whether girls respond to CBT for anger and aggression differently than boys. Interestingly, in our meta-analysis of 40 randomized studies of CBT for anger in adolescents, we found that the percent of girls in a study sample was positively associated with the magnitude of the effect size observed in this study (Sukhodolsky, Kassinove, & Gorman, 2004). In other words, the larger number of girls in the study was associated with better results. In our own clinical work we also find that girls are as likely to show a positive response to CBT for anger and aggression as boys. We include mostly gender-neutral examples in the manual to make it relevant to both genders as well as some examples that come from our experience of using this treatment with girls. However, to avoid the cumbersome use of "he or she" we opted to use "he" throughout the manual because disruptive behavior disorders are more common in boys.

PURPOSE AND STRUCTURE OF THE MANUAL

This book presents a CBT manual for anger and aggression that can be applied as an individually administered psychotherapy. This treatment is geared toward children and adolescents between the ages of 8 and 16 years with significant levels of anger, aggression, and noncompliance. This is the age range for which CBT has been best studied so far. Younger children are more likely to benefit from parent training. CBT approaches for anger that have been developed for adults (Kassinove & Tafrate, 2002) may be more age-appropriate for older adolescents (17 and older). This treatment is not intended for a specific DSM-IV diagnosis, but rather for a range of behavioral problems (anger, aggression, and noncompliance) that may be part of various psychiatric disorders. Anger and noncompliance are the core symptoms of oppositional defiant disorder and are frequently associated features of conduct disorder and ADHD (American Psychiatric Association, 2000). Irritability and explosive outbursts are prominent features of mood disorders (Weisbrot & Ettinger, 2002), anxiety (Bubier & Drabick, 2009), and pervasive developmental disorders (Kraijer, 2000). Diagnostic assessment should be conducted to determine the presence of psychopathology and to determine what treatments may address the target symptoms.

The CBT program presented in this book can be used in conjunction with other concomitant psychosocial or pharmacological treatments for children with multiple co-occurring disorders. It can be also used as a stand-alone treatment for children whose disruptive behavior is the only clinical problem. We note that serious and persistent forms of juvenile delinquency such as weapon violence, drug use, and other criminal behaviors require comprehensive treatments. One example of such treatments, multisystemic therapy (MST), is briefly reviewed below. Outpatient CBT for anger may be one part of broader treatments for serious conduct problems and juvenile delinquency. It should be noted that there are also specific types of conduct problems, such as fire setting, that have specialized, dedicated treatments (Kolko, Herschell, & Scharf, 2006). Finally, children whose anger and aggression co-occur with untreated psychiatric disorders such as ADHD, major depression, or autism may require medication management for these disorders. If after a few months of medication management for the primary psychiatric disorder, anger and aggression remain as significant clinical problems, CBT may be considered for these behavioral problems in addition to medication or other treatments that the child may be receiving for the primary diagnosis.

The manual consists of 10 sessions, which are divided into three modules (anger management, problem solving, and the development of social skills for preventing and resolving conflict situations). The sessions should occur approximately once a week and run for 1 hour. Consecutive sessions contain materials and skills that build on one another, promoting a consistent acquisition of knowledge and skills by the patient. The guidelines for each session begin with a list of six to eight session goals. These goals represent the tasks that should be accomplished by the therapist during that particular session. Each of the session's goals can be accomplished by a subset of possible therapeutic activities. Within each session, all activities are grouped into sections and numbered to correspond to the session's goals. Each activity is first outlined for the therapist and then a sample presentation for the patient is provided in a different typeface. The therapist should not read from the manual during the session but rather should present each activity to the child in his own words so that the process of therapy is natural. However, there are some key points that can be included by the therapists either verbatim or paraphrased from the text. Therapists should select those activities that correspond to the patient's developmental level, cooperation, current concerns, and target disruptive behavior symptoms.

At the end of each session children receive a homework assignment to practice the skills that are discussed during the session. The homework assignment forms are included as part of this manual (see Appendix 1) and can be copied and given to the child at the end of the session. The therapists can also choose to give some of the in-session handouts to children as take-home reminders of the session content. We experimented with asking our patients and study participants to carry a binder with study forms. Some children remember to bring these binders and others consistently forget or lose them. Over time we learned that giving a new paper form each time and enthusiastically praising the child for bringing it back completed at the next session is the most realistic way of keeping track of written assignments, which can be collected and kept in the child's file.

In addition to the 10 child sessions, we include an outline for three 30-minute parent sessions dedicated to collecting information, informing parents about the treatment, and asking parents to encourage their child to practice new skills at home. The first parent session should be conducted prior to the first child session. The second parent session should be conducted at the midpoint of the child's treatment (i.e., before or after Session 5). The third parent session should be conducted before or after the child's final session. Shorter check-ins with the parent should be conducted at the end of each session to review progress and discuss skills covered in session. We also provide a brief description of parent management training (PMT) in the "Treatment Approaches" section of this Introduction, but structured PMT is not part of this manual. Several excellent resources on PMT have been published (Barkley, 1997; Kazdin, 2005; McMahon & Forehand, 2003).

The manual was developed as part of our continuing research on behavioral treatment for children with neuropsychiatric disorders (Scahill et al., 2006; Sukhodolsky & Butter, 2006; Sukhodolsky, Golub, Stone, & Orban, 2005; Sukhodolsky, Kassinove, & Gorman, 2004; Sukhodolsky & Ruchkin, 2006; Sukhodolsky, Solomon, & Perine, 2000; Sukhodolsky et al., 2009). We discuss the rationale and evidence in support of its effectiveness in the sections that follow. Although several excellent resources are available in the field of anger control (Feindler & Ecton, 1986; Kellner, 2001; Lochman, Wells, & Lenhart, 2008), most are written in a group therapy format for use in school or inpatient settings. Our manual has been developed for providing CBT in a format of individual weekly psychotherapy. We hope it will fill an important niche as an evidence-based treatment for anger and aggression that can be provided in the format of individual psychotherapy in outpatient mental health services for children and adolescents. Another feature that sets this book apart is the focus on flexible yet reliable implementation of treatment. We include Treatment Fidelity Checklists (see Appendix 5) to aid in evaluating adherence to the manual, an important part of implementing treatment in a reliable fashion. We also provide guidelines for the flexible implementation of treatment by selecting from several numbered activities within each treatment goal that can be matched to presenting complaints, on the one hand, and to the child's motivation and developmental characteristics, on the other hand.

This treatment manual is intended for clinicians with a background in child psychopathology and behavior therapy. We also hope that it can be used in training programs for psychologists, psychiatrists, social workers, psychiatric nurse practitioners, and other professionals who provide mental health services to children.

RELEVANT MODELS OF ANGER AND AGGRESSION

Three lines of research on anger and aggression provide the foundation for this CBT program. Within the behavioral or learning approach, aggression is conceptualized in terms of reinforcement history. Within the social information-processing approach, aggression is viewed as stemming from cognitive deficits and distortions. The third approach, which focuses on emotional arousal, suggests that aggressive behavior is mediated by angry affect.

The *behavioral or learning model* explains aggression in terms of classical conditioning, operant conditioning, and observational learning. One of the earliest theories, the frustration–aggression hypothesis, posits that aggression always follows situations in which the person's goals are thwarted or blocked (Dollard, Dood, Miller, Mowrer, & Sears, 1939). Correspondingly, aggressive behavior can be either reactive (i.e., classically conditioned responses to frustration) or proactive (i.e., operant behaviors intended to prevent the frustration). In both cases, aggressive behavior is viewed as a function of situational contingencies that evoke learned behavioral reactions. The development of aggression may be maintained by coercive family interactions, which reinforce the child's disruptive behavior through the mechanisms of negative reinforcement (Patterson, Reid, & Dishion, 1992). For example, when parents withdraw limit setting in response to a child's temper tantrum, the tantrum is negatively reinforced by the removal of the unpleasant parental discipline. The advantage of this model is that it provides clear guidance for treatment of well-defined target symptoms. Child-focused therapies that originated within the learning approach use social skills training procedures to replace aggressive behavior with socially acceptable behaviors (Goldstein & Glick, 1987).

The *social-cognitive model* also provides theoretical and empirically supported explanations for the development and maintenance of aggressive behaviors. This model stems from social learning theory (Bandura, 1973) and problem-solving applications to behavior modification (d'Zurilla & Goldfried, 1971). The social information-processing model developed by Dodge (1980) postulated a five-step sequential model of cognitive processes. These steps are encoding of social cues, interpretation of cues, response search, response decision, and enactment of behavior. Disruption of any of these processes can result in aggressive behavior. For example, people get angry when they think that they have been treated unfairly and when they view the unfair treatment as being inflicted upon them on purpose. These thoughts may be triggered not by the actual actions of another person, but by a distorted understanding of intent. This distortion in processing social information, referred to as "hostile attribution bias," often leads to increased anger arousal and aggressive behavior. Correspondingly, cognitive processes implicated in children's aggression have been targeted by social problem-solving interventions (Kazdin, Esveldt-Dawson, French, & Unis, 1987; Shure & Spivack, 1982).

The *emotional arousal model* suggests that physiological arousal and the intensity of angry feelings may be related to overt aggression. For example, Berkowitz's (1990) model of aggression proposes that negative affect and angry feelings mediate hostile aggression. Aggressive children were found to have sharp increases in physiological arousal during provocation, which adversely affected their social problem-solving strategies (Lochman, Whidby, & FitzGerald, 2000). Several studies have also demonstrated a correlation between the levels of anger assessed by self-report with various forms of aggressive behavior (Sukhodolsky & Ruchkin, 2004). Specific therapeutic techniques that directly target physiological arousal, such as progressive muscle relaxation or positive imagery, are commonly included as parts of muticomponent treatments (Hazaleus & Deffenbacher, 1986), but the separate effect of "arousal reduction" techniques on aggressive behavior has not been well studied. To date, only a few studies have examined independent effects of arousal reduction procedures (Garrison & Stolberg, 1983; Goldbeck & Schmid, 2003) on disruptive behavior.

ASSESSMENT

Competent assessment and diagnosis is a necessary step toward selecting and implementing the right treatment. The presence of clinically significant levels of disruptive behavior can warrant delivery of this treatment to children with different psychiatric diagnosis (see above discussion of anger, aggression, and noncompliance as three common targets of this treatment). This section describes several assessment and rating scales that can help clinicians gauge the levels of severity of behavior problems as well as monitor change in disruptive behavior with treatment. The therapists who will administer this treatment may or may not be involved in clinical assessment before the treatment. For example, in clinical research studies, assessments and treatment are commonly provided by different clinicians. Some child mental health clinics may have their own clinical assessments that would be conducted by an intake specialist before the case is assigned to a therapist. In other clinics and in private practice the same clinician may conduct assessment and treatment. Competent diagnostic evaluation is needed to determine whether anger and aggression are clinically significant problems and whether other conditions are present that require treatment. Structured psychiatric interviews are standard in clinical research. We have favored the Schedule for Affective Disorders and Schizophrenia for School-Age Children (K-SADS; Kaufman et al., 1997) in our work. We suggest that clinicians who were not involved in diagnostic assessment (whether in clinical research or clinical practice) review the results of the assessment prior to initiating the treatment with this CBT manual. To make certain that there is a meeting of minds about the nature of the current problem and the treatment, review of the assessment results with the child and family is also warranted.

As an extension of this collaborative treatment enterprise, we have found that eliciting the "parent-nominated target problems" can help guide evaluation and goal setting for treatment (Arnold et al., 2003). During initial evaluation, parents are asked to describe the child's two most pressing disruptive behavioral problems. These target symptoms can be documented according to their frequency (episodes per day or per week), intensity (amplitude, duration, and actual appearance of the behavior), and impact (degree of disruption at home and school). For example, at baseline the target problem "tantrum" could occur three to five times per day, lasting 10 to 30 minutes accompanied by yelling, slamming doors, and threats of harm, with occasional physical aggression or property destruction. Parents may describe conflict avoidance and near constant tension in the home. After the frequency, intensity, and impact of the target problems are identified, the goals of treatment can be designed to reduce these dimensions. At subsequent follow-up assessments, new narratives for the same problem can be created and used to judge progress.

Although a plethora of measures of anger and aggression are available (Collett, Ohan, & Myers, 2003; Eckhardt, Norlander, & Deffenbacher, 2004), none can be considered the "gold standard" at the moment. Furthermore, the expression of disruptive behaviors varies in different contexts. For example, temper tantrums and noncompliance are most likely to occur at home, while covert antisocial behaviors may take place during unsupervised time spent with peers. Consequently, parents, teachers, and children may provide different accounts of disruptive behavior, and researchers may face the challenge of integrating data from multiple informants (Kraemer et al., 2003). Below, we briefly review several instruments that have been used in the ongoing investigations of child disruptive behavior at the Yale Child Study Center.

The *Disruptive Behavior Rating Scale* (DBRS; Barkley, 1997) is an eight-item parent-rated scale keyed to the DSM-IV criteria for oppositional defiant disorder. The parent is asked to rate each item on a 4-point scale, where 0 = never or rarely, 1 = sometimes, 2 = often, and 3 = very often. The internal consistency of the scale ranges from .86 to .93 (Gomez, Burns, & Walsh, 2008), and scores of 12 and higher are considered clinically significant (Barkley, Edwards, Laneri, Fletcher, & Metevia, 2001). This scale has been used as a primary outcome measure in our studies of behavior therapy for disruptive behavior in children and adolescents with Tourette syndrome (Scahill et al., 2006; Sukhodolsky et al., 2009). As with the DBRS, the SNAP-IV ODD scale is also derived from DSM-IV criteria for oppositional defiant disorder. This 10-item scale was used as an outcome measure in the MTA study (MTA Cooperative Group, 1999). Both the DBRS and the SNAP-IV ODD scales can be completed by teachers.

The *Home Situations Questionnaire* (HSQ; Barkley, 1997) is a 16-item measure of noncompliance. Parents are asked to answer *yes* or *no* to items that describe typical situations within which disruptive behavior is likely to occur. Items marked *yes* are then rated on a 1 (mild) to 9 (severe) scale. The HSQ yields two scores: the number of problem situations and the mean severity value (total severity score divided by 16 for the number of items). The scale has normative data (DuPaul & Barkley, 1992) and it has been shown to be sensitive to stimulant-drug effects and to effects of parent management training (Aman et al., 2009). The HSQ can be presented as an interview; a school version of the measure is available. The DBRS and the HSQ are included in Appendices 2 and 3, respectively, and can be used to gauge the levels of disruptive behavior and monitor treatment progress.

The *Child Behavior Checklist* (CBCL; Achenbach, 1991) is a 116-item parent report, which asks the parent to rate overall areas of behavioral and somatic symptoms on a 0 to 2 scale. The CBCL provides national age and gender norms, and an extensive body of research supports the scale's reliability and validity. It features both narrow-band (Aggression and Delinquency) and broad-band (Externalizing problems) factors that are relevant to the evaluation of disruptive behavior. The Aggressive behavior scale consists of 20 items that measure physical aggression, argumentativeness, and excessive anger. The scale has high internal consistency of .92 in both referred and nonreferred children. The Delinquent behavior scale consists of 13 items of antisocial behaviors, including lying, stealing, truancy, vandalism, and drug use. The internal consistency of the scale ranges from .74 to .83 for younger and older children, respectively. The CBCL is probably the most commonly used behavior rating scale and the Aggression subscale is a useful tool for gauging the level of a child's aggressive behavior in comparison to the age and gender-matched standardization group.

The *Overt Aggression Scale* (OAS; Silver & Yudofsky, 1991; Yudofsky, Silver, Jackson, Endicott, & Williams, 1986) is an observer-rated instrument that reflects characteristics and seriousness of incidents of aggressive behavior. The scale consists of four categories of aggression: (1) verbal aggression, (2) aggression against objects, (3) self-directed aggression, and (4) aggression against others. Each category contains four statements describing aggressive behaviors at increasing levels of severity. All statements that apply to a child's behavior during an episode of aggression are checked off by the rater and assigned a weighted score. Verbal aggression is scored on a scale of 1 to 4; aggression against objects, of 2 to 5; and physical aggression against self or others, of 3 to 6. In addition to documenting the occurrence and severity of the four types of aggression, the OAS provides a global measure of aggression severity, calculated as the sum of the weighted scores of the most severe behaviors in each category (range, 0 to 21). The OAS has been shown to have adequate interrater and test–retest reliability coefficients. It has been also shown to be sensitive to change in clinical studies of pharmacological treatments for children with aggressive behavior (Armenteros & Lewis, 2002; Malone, Delaney, Luebbert, Cater, & Campbell, 2000).

The *Aberrant Behavior Checklist* (ABC; Aman, Singh, Stewart, & Field, 1985) is a 58-item, informant-based scale comprising five subscales: *I. Irritability* (includes agitation, aggression, and self-injurious behaviors, 15 items); II. *Lethargy/Social Withdrawal* (16 items); III. *Stereotypic Behaviors* (seven items); IV. *Hyperactivity* (includes noncompliance, 16 items); and V. *Inappropriate Speech* (four items). The ABC has normative values for children with developmental disabilities (Brown, Aman, & Havercamp, 2002). The Irritability subscale, which has been used as an outcome measure in children with autism spectrum disorders, reflects tantrums, aggression, and self-injurious behavior (Aman et al., 2009).

Child self-report may add unique information on aspects of disruptive behavior such as subjective anger experience and covert antisocial behavior. Several instruments with extensive normative information are currently available but only a few have been used in treatment studies. The *Children's Inventory of Anger* (ChIA; Nelson & Finch, 2000) is a 39-item measure of anger intensity in response to hypothetical provoking events (e.g., "Someone cuts in front of you in a lunch line"). The ChIA provides norms for children from 6 to 16 years.

The *State–Trait Anger Expression Inventory* (STAXI; Spielberger, 1988) is a 44-item self-report measure, which contains two scales of experience and three scales of anger expression. The STAXI is one of the most researched psychometric instruments for anger. The first edition of the test provides norms for 12- to 16 year-old children and has been shown to be sensitive to change in anger management training for adolescents (Snyder, Kymissis, Kessler, & Snyder, 1999). The second edition of the STAXI has been recently standardized in a sample of 836 children and adolescents (Brunner & Spielberger, 2009).

TREATMENT APPROACHES

Psychosocial treatments for anger and aggression in children can be focused on children, parents, or broader systems and services. A comprehensive review of these treatment modalities is outside the scope of this book, but a brief summary will help to place this CBT method for anger and aggression in the context of other available treatments. The label "cognitive-behavioral" is used here to reflect a strong emphasis on the learning principles and the use of structured strategies to produce changes in thinking, feeling, and behavior (Kendall, 2006). Although CBT is conducted with the child, parents have multiple roles in treatment, including bringing their child to treatment, providing information, and creating the environment between sessions in which the child can practice the skills learned in treatment.

Child-Focused Treatments

Anger control training (ACT) aims to improve emotion regulation and social-cognitive deficits in aggressive children. Children are taught to monitor their emotional arousal and to use techniques such as relaxation for modulating elevated levels of anger experience. As part of the training, children also practice socially appropriate responses to anger-provoking situations such as being teased by peers or reprimanded by adults. ACT was first developed for adults by Novaco (1975), based on Meichenbaum's stress inoculation model (Meichenbaum & Cameron, 1973). Several programs of research have evaluated versions of anger control training with children (Lochman, Barry, & Pardini, 2003), adolescents (Deffenbacher, Lynch, Oetting, & Kemper, 1996; Feindler & Ecton, 1986), and adults (DiGuiseppe & Tafrate, 2003; Kassinove & Tafrate, 2002).

Problem-solving skills training (PSST) addresses cognitive processes, such as faulty perception and decision making, that are involved in social interaction. For example, hostile attribution bias or inability to generate alternative solutions may contribute to aggressive behavior. Beginning from research on social information processing (Dodge, Bates, & Pettit, 1990) and problem solving in children (Shure & Spivack, 1972), scores of studies have examined the association between thinking in social situations and aggressive behavior (Dodge, 2003). Over the past three decades several PSST approaches were developed for use by mental health and education specialists to help adolescents cope with interpersonal conflicts. Modifications of this treatment approach are available for young children (Shure, 1993), incarcerated juveniles (Bourke & Van Hasselt, 2001), and adults (D'Zurilla & Goldfried, 1971). Participants in PSST are taught to analyze interpersonal conflicts, to develop nonaggressive solutions, and to think about the consequences of their actions in problematic situations. The efficacy of PSST has been demonstrated in several controlled studies (Guerra & Slaby, 1990; Hudley & Graham, 1993; Kazdin, Siegel, & Bass, 1992). Initial evidence indicates that the effects of PSST on conduct problems may be mediated by change in the targeted deficits in social information processing (Sukhodolsky et al., 2005).

Social skills training (SST) has been part of the treatment program for various disorders including schizophrenia and autism, as well as for disruptive behavior problems in children. As a result, the actual skills taught during a particular program may be different depending on the clinical population. The techniques used in SST, however, are similar across disorders. These techniques involve modeling, role play, corrective feedback, and reinforcement for appropriate performance (Merrell & Gimpel, 1998; Spence, 2003). SST programs are based on the assumption that socially acceptable behavior can be enhanced through these training procedures. The theoretical background of SST can be traced to social learning theory (Bandura, 1973), as well as to early behavioral approaches to psychotherapy (Wolpe, 1958). Aggressive youth have been shown to have weak verbal skills, poor conflict resolution skills, and deficits in skills that facilitate friendships (Barratt, Kent, Felthous, & Stanford, 1997; Deater-Deckard, 2001). The goal of SST with aggressive youth is to enhance or develop specific social behaviors that can be deployed instead of aggression, as well as behaviors that can be used to develop friendships with nondelinquent peers. Several narrative and meta-analytic reviews of SST with children and adolescents are available with estimated moderate effect on reduction of antisocial behavior (Losel & Beelmann, 2003).

Family- and Community-Focused Treatments

The beneficial effects of youth-focused treatments on mild to moderate forms of disruptive behavior have been well documented. However, serious and chronic conduct problems as well as juvenile delinquency are likely to require more intensive services and include a broader range of systems. Family-based programs target family risk factors for child disruptive behavior including inconsistent or harsh discipline and poor supervision.

Parent management training (PMT) is a psychosocial treatment in which parents are taught skills for managing their children's disruptive behavior (Kazdin, 2005). The broad goals of PMT are to improve parental competence in dealing with the child's maladaptive behavior and to improve the child's adaptive behavior. PMT teaches parents to identify the function of maladaptive behavior, to give praise for appropriate behavior, to communicate directions effectively, to ignore maladaptive attention-seeking behavior, and to use consistent consequences for disruptive behaviors. New parenting skills are developed through modeling, practice, role play, and feedback. PMT techniques stem from the fundamental principle of operant conditioning, which states that the likelihood of behavior to recur is increased or weakened based on the events that follow the behavior (Skinner, 1938). For example, a child is more likely to have another tantrum if previous tantrums have led to escape from parental demand or continuation of a preferred activity. Furthermore, PMT targets those parent–child interactions that have been shown to foster disruptive behaviors. Behaviors such as noncompliance, whining, or bickering can be reinforced if they result in escape or avoidance of situations such as homework or room cleaning that could be aversive to the child (Patterson, DeBaryshe, & Ramsey, 1989). Harsh and inconsistent discipline such as excessive scolding and corporal punishment have also been shown to increase a child's aggression (Gershoff, 2002). PMT has been evaluated in over 100 randomized controlled studies, and several programs of research in different centers continue to investigate this treatment. There is evidence that the improvements in child behavior are stable over time and can improve other areas such as reduction in family stress (Webster-Stratton, Hollinsworth, & Kolpacoff, 1989).

Multisystemic therapy (MST) is based on socioecological (Bronfenbrenner, 1979) and family systems (Minuchin, 1974) models of behavior. It targets multiple individual, family, peer, school, and community risk factors for delinquency. MST shares common characteristics with traditional family therapies, but also includes problem-focused interventions that address specific areas within peer, school, and other systems as needed. Treatment is usually delivered over a 3- to 5-month period by a team of master's-level counselors who are trained and supervised in MST techniques. Most sessions are conducted in the home at a convenient time for the family, but some meetings are held in other locations, such as schools or community mental health centers. Because treatment is highly individualized, the frequency and number of sessions may vary among participants. For example, in the two primary outcome studies of MST (Borduin et al., 1995; Henggeler, Melton, & Smith, 1992), the duration of direct contact was 33 (*SD* = 29) and 24 (*SD* = 8) hours. Treatment manuals and procedures for training, supervision, and monitoring of treatment fidelity are available and provide guidance on flexible delivery of the treatment. The effects of MST on delinquent behavior have been evaluated in several randomized controlled studies (Borduin et al., 1995; Henggeler et al., 1992; Henggeler, Pickrel, & Brondino, 1999; Henggeler, Rowland, et al., 1999). A long-term follow-up demonstrated that delinquent youth who received MST had lower rearrest rates and shorter incarceration periods compared to youth in the usual treatment condition (Schaeffer & Borduin, 2005).

Medication Management

In addition to psychosocial interventions for disruptive behavior such as anger and aggression, various medications have also been evaluated for these target problems. Although there is variability in the state of the evidence, the list of medications studied includes the atypical antipsychotics, stimulants, and mood stabilizers. Interest in the atypical antipsychotics emerged from the promise of efficacy and a better side effect profile than the traditional antipsychotics (Jensen et al., 2003; Schur et al., 2003). The atypical antipsychotics include clozapine, risperidone, olanzapine, quetiapine, ziprasidone, and aripiprazole. Of these, risperidone is the best studied. Target problems described as disruptive behavior, explosiveness, aggression, or all of these have been evaluated in children with autism spectrum disorders (RUPP Autism Network, 2002) and shown positive effects. Weight gain has emerged as a potential adverse effect. Other drugs in this class have been less well studied, but may also have adverse effects. Therefore, the use of these medications for disruptive and explosive behavior is usually reserved for children with serious aggressive behavior. Stimulant medications such as methylphenidate have been shown to reduce symptoms of oppositional defiant disorder in children with ADHD (MTA Cooperative Group, 1999). Other classes of drugs used in the treatment of aggressive and disruptive behavior include anticonvulsants and lithium. Although there are some encouraging results for divalproex (Donovan et al., 2000) and lithium (Malone et al., 2000), these mood stabilizers require close monitoring and may also have adverse effects.

EFFECTIVENESS OF CBT FOR ANGER AND AGGRESSION

Several randomized studies have evaluated CBT for anger and aggression in children (Lochman et al., 2003; Sukhodolsky et al., 2000) and adolescents (Deffenbacher et al., 1996; Feindler & Ecton, 1986; Snyder et al., 1999; Sukhodolsky et al., 2009).

In one of the early studies, John Lochman evaluated a 12-session, group, cognitive-behavioral intervention with 76 elementary school children who were rated by teachers as highly aggressive (Lochman, Curry, Burch, & Lampron, 1984). The active treatment consisted of teaching anger coping, social problem-solving, and goal-setting skills and resulted in reduction of disruptive behavior in school and at home. This school-based anger-coping program has become a segment of a multicomponent Coping Power Program that has received extensive support within a program of conduct problems prevention research (Lochman & Wells, 2004; Lochman et al., 2008).

Feindler evaluated cognitive-behavioral anger control training in adolescents. One study was conducted with 36 adolescents who attended a school-based program for students with disruptive behavior. Compared to the waiting-list control group, adolescents who received the treatment demonstrated significant improvement on self-report measures of self-control and social problem solving. In addition, significant improvement was observed in the number of staff-recorded episodes of disruptive behavior (Feindler, Marriott, & Iwata, 1984). A second study investigated anger control training in a sample of 21 male adolescents hospitalized in a psychiatric facility. Compared to the waiting-list control group, adolescents who received active treatment were rated as significantly less aggressive by staff members (Feindler, Ecton, Kingsley, & Dubey, 1986). In our meta-analysis of 40 studies of CBT for youth with disruptive behavior (Sukhodolsky et al., 2004), the overall effect size was in the high medium range (Cohen's $d = 0.67$) and consistent with the effectiveness of psychotherapy with children in general (Weisz & Weiss, 1993).

Our own clinical research on the effectiveness of CBT for anger and aggression has been conducted over the past 10 years. The first study evaluated a 10-session group CBT training in 33 elementary school children who were referred by teachers for anger-related problems (Sukhodolsky et al., 2000). Compared to the no-treatment control condition, the treatment group displayed a reduction on teacher reports of aggressive and disruptive behavior and improvement on self-reported anger control. In the second study we investigated the relative effectiveness of the social skills training and problem-solving training components of CBT (Sukhodolsky et al., 2005). Twenty-six children were referred by their parents for high levels of disruptive behavior and randomized to one of two treatments. The first treatment, social skills training, included modeling, behavioral rehearsal, and corrective feedback aimed at the development of socially appropriate ways of dealing with interpersonal conflicts. The second treatment, problem-solving training, provided cognitive restructuring, attribution retraining, and solution generation that targeted social-cognitive deficits implicated in anger and aggression. Parent ratings of aggression and conduct problems indicated that both treatments resulted in significant improvements with no differences between groups on child self-report measures. The problem-solving condition resulted in greater improvement in the hostile attribution bias; the skills-training condition resulted in greater improvement in the anger-control skills.

The treatment described in this book was also evaluated in our study of CBT for anger and aggression in adolescents with Tourette syndrome complicated by disruptive behavior. Although Tourette syndrome is diagnosed based on the presence of unwanted movements and vocalizations called "tics," many children with Tourette syndrome have co-occurring behavioral problems such as anger outbursts and non-compliance. Because CBT has been shown to reduce disruptive behavior in children without tics, we evaluated this treatment in children with tics and co-occurring disruptive behavior. The study included 26 adolescents with Tourette syndrome and disruptive behavior who were randomized to receive CBT or to continue with treatment as usual. Children received 10 weekly individual CBT sessions. Assessments, which included evaluations by a blinded rater, parent reports, and child self-reports, were conducted before and after treatment as well as 3 months posttreatment. All randomized subjects completed endpoint evaluation. The parent rating of disruptive behavior decreased by 52% in the CBT condition compared with a decrease of 11% in the control condition. The independent evaluator who was unaware of treatment assignment rated nine of 13 subjects (69%) in the CBT condition as much improved or very much improved compared with two of 13 (15%) in the control condition. This reduction of disruptive behavior in the CBT group was statistically significant and well maintained at 3-month follow-up. To our knowledge, this is one of the few studies that investigated individually (rather than group-) administered CBT for anger and aggression. Indeed, in preparation for developing the treatment manual used in our study of adolescents with Tourette syndrome, we found that nearly all manuals used a group format. Thus, we concluded that a CBT manual for an individual treatment of anger and aggression would be useful for clinicians and investigators.

ADHERENCE TO THE MANUAL AND TREATMENT FIDELITY

The advent of treatment manuals has been referred to as a "small revolution" in psychotherapy research (Luborsky & DeRubeis, 1984), and currently they are considered a requirement for clinical trials. Virtually all psychosocial treatments for children that have achieved a status of evidence-based interventions include detailed manuals, and procedures for constructing and delivering treatment manuals have been outlined (Perepletchikova & Kazdin, 2005). From the standpoint of methodology, the availability of manuals in randomized clinical trails (experiments) is a prerequisite for being able to confirm that the treatment (independent variable) was delivered as planned (has internal validity). There is evidence that greater treatment fidelity can be related to better clinical outcomes in treatments for conduct problems (Henggeler, Brondino, Melton, Scherer, & Hanley, 1997). In order to help clinicians monitor treatment fidelity (adherence to the treatment manual), we have included the Treatment Fidelity Checklist (see Appendix 5) that was used in our research. The items on this checklist match with the goals of each session and are rated on a 0 to 2 scale anchored to poor, partial, and complete attainment of a session goal. As a rule of thumb, 80% fidelity is considered adequate in clinical research studies. Through the use of the fidelity checklist, clinicians can evaluate their own performance in the delivery of the manual.

Guidelines for Flexible Implementation

Of course, rigid delivery of treatment, such as reading long sections of the manual during the session or pursuing topics that are part of the manual but clearly irrelevant to a particular child, is the fastest way to a no-show the following week. Flexibility within fidelity is an important consideration for a competent administration of any manualized treatment (Kendall, Chu, Gifford, Hayes, & Nauta, 1998). We suggest that therapists administer all 10 sessions and strive to accomplish session goals. However, within each session, the goals can be attained by a variety of techniques and activities that allow for a flexible implementation of the treatment. Within each session, activities are grouped into sections and numbered to correspond to the session's goals. Each activity is outlined for the therapist and followed by a sample script for the patient that is presented in another typeface. These scripts are not intended to be read during the session. Therapists are encouraged to become familiar with the content of the script and then to use their own words to communicate in a natural, conversational manner.

The flexible application of the manual implies that some portions of the manual may not be relevant to all patients. Based on the patient's development, level of cooperation, current concerns, and target disruptive behaviors, the therapist may select some activities over others. For example, we have found that only a few participants in our studies on CBT were interested in progressive muscle relaxation. Thus, we include the description of progressive muscle relaxation as an optional technique in this manual. To maintain treatment fidelity, however, the therapist should aim to address all treatment goals by selecting age-appropriate activities within each goal category. We also encourage therapists to be creative in their delivery of the treatment but only after the core techniques of the manual have been covered. For example, a mother of one of our recent patients was a yoga instructor with experience teaching yoga to children. She knew various engaging exercises to help focus on breathing, such as keeping a light feather in the air by blowing at it. We asked that she try these breathing exercises with her son instead of deep breathing relaxation. Flexible implementation of the manual should be guided by clinical skills and experience. Experienced therapists can use their clinical judgment to select or modify activities within each session and goal category. Therapists in training should seek supervision as they administer this treatment with their first two or three children.

MODULE 1

ANGER MANAGEMENT

Introduction to CBT and Education about Anger

★ **GOALS**

1. Present the rationale for treatment.
2. Review treatment goals.
3. Define anger and the elements of anger episodes.
4. Discuss the child's typical anger-provoking situations.
5. Discuss the frequency, intensity, and duration of recent anger episodes.
6. Discuss typical coping responses and introduce distraction and brief relaxation.
7. Summarize the session and assign homework.
8. Check in with parent(s).

 HANDOUTS

Disruptive Behavior Rating Scale (DBRS) (for parents)
Home Situations Questionnaire (HSQ) (for parents)
Elements of an Anger Episode
Anger Triggers
Distract Yourself from Anger

☑ **HOMEWORK**

Daily Anger Monitoring Log (optional)
Anger Management Log 1

If the therapist has not been involved in the preliminary assessment, as discussed in the Introduction, the first session will be the time when the therapist and the child get to know each other and establish a rapport, with the main objective being to gain the child's commitment to the program. Therapists may also ask the parent to complete the **Disruptive Behavior Rating Scale** and the **Home Situations Questionnaire** before the first session to evaluate the child's current levels of anger and noncompliance. This manual contains the outline for three 30-minute parent sessions. The first parent session should be conducted before the first child session; the other two parent sessions can be scheduled in the middle and at the end of treatment, either before or after child sessions. Guidelines for parent sessions are provided at the end of this manual.

1.   ***Present the rationale for treatment.*** The rationale for treatment can be introduced in a number of different ways depending on the participant's age, motivation, and degree of cooperation. Usually, children referred for this or similar programs would acknowledge having problems with anger or admit to getting into fights and arguments with friends, parents, and teachers. If this is the case, the rationale for treatment can be presented in a simple manner:

Everyone gets angry every now and then. Anger is a normal emotion that tells us if something is not going our way. People get angry if they don't get what they want, if they are bossed around, or if they are insulted or offended. However, sometimes people get angry for the wrong reasons or express their anger inappropriately. If we lose control over what we are saying or doing because of anger, it can create all kinds of problems for us and for other people. This program has been used for many years to teach young people, like you, about different strategies for anger management.

1.1.   It can be helpful to *provide a few general facts about anger in daily life.* For example, therapists can say that on average people experience anger at least once a week and that it lasts for approximately half an hour. Most of the time people get angry when they are at home as opposed to other places. Interestingly, most of the time people report being angry at someone they love as opposed to someone they dislike. People often get angry if they are tired, hungry, or already in a bad mood. The medical consequences of excessive anger include high blood pressure and increased risk of cardiac problems.

1.2.   If the child is cooperative and eager to share his personal experiences, the therapist might *ask about specific situations that could make the child angry or lead to conflicts.* For children who are more reserved or need more time to become engaged in a conversation, it can be helpful to talk about some neutral topics such as hobbies, interests, or sports before proceeding to discussion of the treatment.

1.3.   It is helpful to *be flexible with the choice of words* because, for various reasons, some children may not admit to getting angry too much or too frequently. For example, some children may not want to be in therapy or talk about their feelings. If this seems to be the case, the therapist might frame the purpose of treatment in terms of problem solving. We have also worked with children who did not like to use the word *angry*, preferring instead words such as *frustrated* or *upset*. It is preferable to use the language suggested by the participant for anger-provoking events as well as everyday problems. Some of the possible ways to ask about what makes a person angry are as follows:

So what kinds of things make you angry or upset?
How do you feel when your parents tell you to clean your room when you're in the middle of a game?
What happens when you have too much homework?

2.   ***Review treatment goals.*** Because CBT is a short-term structured program, the therapeutic alliance can be viewed as an agreement between the therapist and the child regarding the goals of the treatment. It is likely that children are brought to this program by their parents and may not feel very enthusiastic about sitting and talking to a stranger. If a child can give a few examples of what makes him angry or upset, the best way to define the goal of treatment is to figure out ways to make this type of situation less likely to occur.

This is also a good time to discuss the format of the program: 10 weekly sessions conducted one-on-one with the child. Parents are invited to review presenting concerns and treatment progress at least a few times during the program. It is also helpful to have 10- to 15-minute check-ins with the parent at the end of each session so that the child can tell the parent about what he learned and that they can agree about practicing a particular "anger management" skill during the following week at home.

2.1.   There are *two treatment goals*: (1) to reduce the frequency and intensity of angry and aggressive behaviors, and (2) to increase the child's skills for dealing with conflicts with peers and adults. The following script can be used to present these treatment goals to the child:

There are two goals that we will try to achieve during our visits. First, we want to reduce the number of times you get angry or upset. Being angry does not feel good. I am sure you'd rather feel happy or calm. In this program we will talk about the kinds of things that make you angry and try to see how to prevent them from happening. Our main goal is to reduce the number of times, for example, per week, that you feel angry. Let's say you get angry 10 times per week; we can aim to reduce this number to five times per week. The second goal is to practice different skills and strategies that you might use to solve problems and conflicts in your life—for example, how to discuss things with your teacher if he is treating you unfairly.

2.2.   *Ask the child if he may have any particular reasons to be in the program.* Some common answers are "My parents brought me here" and "I don't know," but children are also likely to acknowledge having arguments with parents or fights with siblings or schoolmates.

The child may be less than enthusiastic about being in the program. If that is the case, more time should be spent on building the therapeutic alliance and helping the child to develop appropriate motivation for being in the program. In this case, the therapist may go beyond the procedures in this manual and use his or her own clinical skills to engage the child in treatment. Parents may be asked to come up with specific rewards to encourage participation in therapy and practice of anger management skills between sessions. This discussion can be part of the parent check-in at the end of the session.

3.   ***Define anger and the elements of anger episodes.*** One way to define anger is by asking the child to tell about a time when he was really angry. Then ask the child how he knows that it was anger, not another emotion such as sadness or fear. Younger children may have a simple response such as "Anger is when you are mad." Older children may engage in a detailed discussion. The important outcome of this activity is that the child and the therapist reach a common understanding of feelings and thoughts that arise in response to frustration or provocation.

3.1.   In addition to examples, a therapist may *use metaphors to illustrate various aspects of anger.* For example, "short fuse" is a metaphor that can be used to describe someone who gets angry quickly. Feindler and Ecton (1986) compared anger to a firecracker and the anger trigger to a match to illustrate how negative thoughts and physiological reactions can contribute to explosive anger outbursts. Then our ability to control anger can be compared to putting out the fuse of the firecracker before it explodes by controlling negative thoughts and feelings.

One participant in this program told us that "anger is like a cartoon with steam coming out of your ears." The therapist proceeded to draw a picture of an angry person with steam coming out of his ears and the child observed that the steam clouds looked like broccoli. We proceeded to refer to anger as "when you feel like broccoli are coming out of your ears." Later, this metaphor led to a discussion of humor as a way of diffusing angry feelings.

3.2.   *Discuss the elements of an anger episode*: triggers, experiences, expressions, and outcomes. The **Elements of an Anger Episode** handout can be used to convey the multicomponential nature of anger. Each element can be discussed either at length or briefly, depending on time and the child's level of interest.

Anger can be triggered by various events such as the actions of other people (e.g., parents say no) and even inanimate objects (e.g., car does not start). This treatment is dedicated to increasing a child's ability to identify and prevent anger-triggering events. The second component of an anger episode is the actual experience of anger as a feeling state. This feeling may be accompanied and even exaggerated by thoughts (e.g., "I really hate this") and physiological reactions (e.g., racing heart). This treatment will teach modulation of the thoughts and sensations that may lead to increased anger and will also teach coping skills to decrease excessive anger. The third element of anger episodes is expressions: display rules and behaviors. For example, facial expressions of anger may include clenched teeth or lowered eyebrows. There are also cultural rules for expressing anger to other people. For example, raising your voice at parents when angry is more likely to occur in some cultures than in others. Finally, there is an outcome to each anger episode that may make the next episode of anger either less or more likely to occur. For example, if yelling and screaming leads to getting one's way, these behaviors will be reinforced and more likely to be repeated.

4.   ***Discuss the child's typical anger-provoking situations.*** Use the **Anger Triggers** handout and ask the child to list five things that usually make him angry. Then group the typical anger triggers into categories. These categories will vary for different participants but may include specific people and actions. For example, consider the following list:

> Being teased or bothered by peers at school.
> Being told to do something by parents in the middle of enjoyable activities.
> Being treated unfairly by a teacher.

The purpose of this activity is to help the child think about the causes of his anger.

4.1.   *Talking about events that provoke anger is usually easier than discussing associated thoughts and feelings.* One reason for this is that people are usually aware of the causes of their anger. It is easier to gain the child's cooperation if the goals of the treatments are defined in terms of preventing anger-provoking situations from occurring. Ask the child to select two situations that frequently make him angry or frustrated. Have a discussion about what he thinks causes these situations and if he has ever tried doing anything to prevent these situations from occurring.

5.   ***Discuss the frequency, intensity, and duration of recent anger episodes.*** Children may underreport the frequency and intensity of their anger episodes compared to their parents. However, self-reported information is central for the child-focused intervention. Therefore, it is important to obtain information about the frequency and duration of typical anger episodes. The **Anger Management Log 1** handout, *which will be assigned as homework,* could be used to help the child recall and describe a recent anger episode. Below is a situation described by one of the participants in the program:

Describe this situation:	I had a detention and I was riding the late bus and the driver went right by my house first thing but then dropped me off last.
Who was involved?	Me.
What did you say?	Nothing, but I was really angry inside.
What did you do?	I sat there with thoughts going through my mind and just stared out the window.

What happened after?	I got off the bus and went inside and did homework and tried not to get mad.	
Is there anything that you could have done differently?	Asked to get off when the driver passed my house.	
Day 11/28	Time 4:00–5:00	Location On the bus

5.1. After typical triggers and anger episodes are described, *the goals of the program can be specified and reformulated in terms that are more relevant to the child's anger contents.* For example, the therapist could say:

We have discussed various things that make you angry and the ways in which you experience anger. The goal of our program is to reduce the frequency of these unpleasant anger feelings. This can be accomplished through increasing your power to control these situations as well as improving your skills to manage anger. For example, the boy who was angry when the bus driver went right by his house without stopping could have taken a deep breath and said to himself, "Well, this is annoying but I'm not gonna worry about it." After that he could have thought instead about something fun to do when he got home.

6. ***Discuss typical coping responses and introduce distraction and brief relaxation.*** Ask the child what he usually does to reduce his anger. Therapists should not be surprised to hear responses such as "I might break or throw something" and "I just punch him in the face." These responses are common and reflective of an erroneous belief that physical aggression reduces anger. The therapist can remind the child that the question was "What do you do to reduce anger?" If the answers are indicative of responses that actually bring anger to the level of physical aggression or disruptive behavior, this could be a good time to identify and dispute beliefs supporting anger and aggression. Examples of such beliefs are:

Expressing anger results in reducing anger intensity.
Punching a pillow (punching a wall, kicking furniture) helps to reduce anger.
If someone makes you angry, he must be punished.
People who do mean things to you should not get away with it.

Most of the time, children agree that verbal arguments and physical aggression actually result in increased feelings of anger. The next logical step is to conclude that a good way of reducing the unpleasant feelings of anger is to avoid escalations.

6.1. *Introduce distraction.* After discussing behaviors that actually increase rather than decrease anger, introduce adaptive (helpful) coping responses. The simplest coping mechanism is to do something enjoyable, such as listening to music, spending time with friends, or playing sports. These enjoyable activities can provide a distraction from feeling angry and frustrated.

Use the **Distract Yourself from Anger** handout, and ask the child to write down several activities in which he might engage in order to reduce his anger. Discuss how likely it is that the child will be able to use each of the proposed activities in his daily schedule, focusing on those activities that the child identifies as the ones he would be most likely to use. Summarize the role of distraction in reducing anger in the following way:

One way to stop being angry is to take your mind off the thing that made you angry. Sometimes just by doing something enjoyable or fun and by letting a few minutes pass, people will feel less angry or frustrated. Reading a book, calling a friend, or simply going for a walk are some good examples of what can be done to distract oneself from being angry. Of course, there is more to this program than just listening to music, but this can be a very useful strategy for bringing down one's anger.

6.2. *Introduce deep breathing relaxation.* A simple way to relax is to breathe rhythmically, deeply, and fully. Model how to properly take a deep breath in front of the child, and then ask the child to practice the technique. The following explanation can be provided.

Place one hand on your stomach and breathe in through your nose and out through your mouth. When the bottoms of your lungs completely fill with air, your hand should move outward. Don't lift your shoulders; imagine the air is flowing into your stomach. When you exhale, your hand should move inward. Close your eyes and practice this exercise for 2 minutes or so.

Let the child practice the breathing exercise and provide feedback, if needed, on the pace and form of inhaling and exhaling.

7. ***Summarize the session and assign homework.*** Each session should end with a summary and a take-home message. The first session is rich with new information, so the therapist should highlight selected topics that resonated with the child. Taking a common or ongoing anger-provoking situation and formulating a coping strategy that would help to improve this situation during the next week can enhance the child's motivation for treatment. We found that distraction and rhythmic breathing relaxation are the easiest anger management techniques for children to learn, and most children who participated in this program with us were able to make use of them. The following script can be used to provide a session summary.

Today we spoke about [summarize an anger-provoking situation reported by the child]. Do you think you will be able to use any of the material that we covered today to handle this situation better?

Let's say the child agrees that going to his room and listening to his favorite music will make him feel better.

OK, so if this or a similar situation happens next week, could you try and practice this strategy at home? You told me that last time it happened, you ended up in an argument and were upset for half an hour. This time, try to go to your room and listen to music, and see if you can calm down in less than half an hour.

7.1. *Practicing anger management skills between sessions is a crucial part of treatment.* These skills can be practiced in naturalistic ways every time an opportunity presents itself and also as formal homework assignments. Written homework assignments are important to increase the chances that the child will think about and practice new skills between the sessions. The scope of homework assignments should also be proportionate to the child's motivation and cooperation. Clinicians should use their judgment and not overload the child with assignments that have low likelihood of being completed.

7.2. **Daily Anger Monitoring Logs** can be used for the first 2 weeks of the program with highly motivated children. The level of motivation can be inferred from cooperation with various tasks of the session as well as general enthusiasm about the treatment. The therapist should ask the child to record and briefly describe all incidents of anger that occur between this session and the next. The therapist and the child should look over the handout and discuss its categories.

7.3. **Anger Management Log 1** should be handed out at the end of this session and completed as homework before the next session. In this assignment, the child is asked to record one episode during that week when he was able to use one of the anger-control techniques effectively. The rationale for this assignment is twofold. First, having this homework assignment serves as a reminder to use anger management techniques in real life. Second, asking the child to describe a situation in which he was able to successfully manage his anger may lead to increased self-efficacy, a belief that he can control his anger.

8. ***Check in with parent(s).*** Because the first session contains a parent component at the beginning, a parent check-in at the end of the session can be relatively brief. At the end of this session, parent(s) or guardian(s) can be invited to review material of the session and the anger management plan for the next week. Ask the child to tell his parents what he learned in session. If needed, therapists may provide two or three bullet points from the session material that resonated most with the child. As noted in Section 2.2, parents can be enlisted to come up with specific rewards to encourage their child to participate in therapy and practice anger management skills between sessions.

Self-Instruction and Relaxation

 GOALS

1. Collect homework and review the last session's material.
2. Discuss anger intensity and the Feeling Thermometer technique.
3. Introduce the Stop & Think technique.
4. Discuss and practice using verbal reminders.
5. Discuss verbal labels for angry feelings.
6. Continue relaxation training.
7. Summarize the session and assign homework.
8. Check in with parent(s).

 MATERIALS

Index cards

 HANDOUTS

Feeling Thermometer
Stop Sign
Words for Anger

 HOMEWORK

Relaxation Practice Log 1
Daily Anger Monitoring Log (optional)
Anger Management Log 2

1.   ***Collect homework and review the last session's material.*** If the child brings completed homework, make sure to thank him and discuss the situation described in **Anger Management Log 1.** If the child fails to complete the homework, ask about the reasons and stress the importance of completing the exercise. Take a few minutes to ask about other anger episodes of the past week.

1.1. *Ask the child to recall the contents of the previous session.* If needed, summarize the last session by saying:

> Last week we spoke about various situations that make people angry and we also listed several situations that typically make you angry. Then we spoke about the elements of an anger response: triggers, feelings and thoughts, behaviors, and consequences. We also discussed how distracting oneself from angry feelings and doing something enjoyable, such as listening to music, may reduce anger and prevent you from doing something that could result in negative consequences. Then we talked about using deep breathing to reduce anger. Were you able to use either distraction or breathing techniques to cope with anger?

2.   ***Discuss anger intensity and the Feeling Thermometer technique.*** The main topic of this session is the intensity of an anger experience. Just like any emotion, anger varies in intensity or strength, and being able to discriminate among various levels of anger intensity is an important part of this treatment. The question of how angry a person feels may be hard to answer. There are psychometric scales such as the state-anger scale of the Spielberger's State–Trait Anger Expression Inventory that attempt to gauge the intensity of one person's anger by comparing his answers to the answers of a large group of people on the standardization sample. The Subjective Units of Distress Scale is commonly used in CBT to rate the intensity of a particular emotional state on a 0 to 10 scale. In our experience, we find a 5-point scale with "discomfort, annoyance, frustration, anger, and rage" as the verbal anchors to provide sufficient range for labeling the intensity of most anger experiences.

The **Feeling Thermometer** handout provides a visual representation of this scale and can be a good starting point to a discussion about various levels of anger intensity. Hot temperature is a natural analogy for anger. Interestingly, there are also research studies that show the link between hot weather and people's anger—very hot days are associated with an increase in the number of fights in the streets.

The **Feeling Thermometer** handout can be used to educate the child about the intensity of emotions as well as using emotion regulation as a way of "dialing down" the intensity of emotion. Ask the child to give examples of situations that would make him feel varying degrees of anger and then ask him to come up with some ideas on how to control these different levels of anger. Lead the discussion to the conclusion that mild levels of anger such as discomfort and annoyance can be ignored; moderate levels of anger such as frustration can be handled by changing your thinking and using relaxation strategies; and intense or explosive levels of anger sometimes labeled as rage are best dealt with by problem solving and prevention.

Ask the child to write down what he can do to reduce each of the five levels of anger intensity and to prevent escalation to the next level on the right-hand side of the handout in the column called "control." For example, a 15-year-old young man who participated in this program wrote the following:

Discomfort—there is always discomfort, if you start thinking about it.
Annoyance—keep in mind, life is too short to worry about it.
Frustration—don't let small stuff bring you down.
Anger—consider other side of the story, what really happened there.
Rage—picture how something very bad may happen.

2.1. *Highlight the importance of monitoring anger intensity.*

Sometimes people go from calm to extremely angry in very fast and even explosive ways. In cases like this, people have difficulty monitoring the moderate levels of anger intensity. If you keep an eye on how your anger is rising, you can do something to prevent it from going through the roof.

If time permits, the therapist can demonstrate how self-focused attention increases body temperature. Similar to the procedures used for progressive muscle relaxation, ask the child to concentrate on the tips of his fingers and imagine the blood flowing to his hands. After a few seconds, ask if he feels how his palms are getting warmer. The parallel may then be drawn that if we can control our body temperature with the power of our mind, we can also control the intensity of angry feelings.

3. ***Introduce the Stop & Think technique.*** It is almost certain that the child can recall a situation when he was angry and did something that he either regretted or that resulted in a negative consequence. A good way to introduce the Stop & Think technique as a way to delay one's response when provoked is to use one of the situations the child described in which he did not act in the best possible way. Visualizing a stop sign and counting to three are the two simple ways to implement the Stop & Think technique.

Unfortunately, we don't always do the right thing when we have a problem with another person. A lot of times we make mistakes. As a matter of fact, no one is perfect and we all make mistakes. One of the reasons that we don't act in our best interest when we are angry is because anger clouds our thinking. As a result when we are angry we don't do what we know is best. Instead, we automatically, that is, without thinking, act in some unfortunate manner. One of the best anger management techniques is called the Stop & Think technique.

Use the **Stop Sign** handout to help the child visualize the stop sign. This visualization technique can be used to delay impulsive response when anger. One of our study participants suggested a variant of this technique that can be useful, particularly for adolescents. He said, "Try to visualize yourself in the back of a police car. It is much more effective."

3.1.   *Provide examples of what can happen when people act without thinking.*

One day, I was waiting to help my student with an assignment. We agreed to meet at 4:00 on Friday afternoon. The student was late, and as the time passed by I got very impatient. I still had some things to do around the office, though, so I continued to wait. However, I would much rather have gone home to start my weekend. Finally, at around 5:00 when the student finally showed up, I almost screamed, "What time is it? When were we supposed to meet? I have been waiting for an hour!" Contrary to my expectations, the student looked confused rather than guilty. "I thought we were supposed to meet at 5:00," he said. Only at this point did I check my calendar and see that the meeting had, in fact, been scheduled for 5:00 P.M. I felt embarrassed and had to apologize.

Misunderstandings happen to children as well. Imagine a child who is playing with other children in the gym, and then what started as a game turns into a squabble. He tries to escape by climbing onto the bleachers. At this point, the gym teacher comes to break up what looks like a fight, and he reaches for the boy to help him down from the bleachers. The boy, however, still thinking he's being chased by the same guys who had been teasing him, kicks back without looking and actually kicks the teacher in the face. Because of his mistake, the boy might end up being blamed for the whole situation.

3.2.   After presenting a few examples, ask the child if he has ever acted without thinking and gotten into trouble as a result. After that, *model the "counting to three" technique.*

When we act without thinking, we get into trouble. A good thing to do is to let some time pass before you do anything when you feel really angry. You can visualize a stop sign as one way of delaying your response. Sometimes letting even 3 seconds pass is enough time to prevent a mistake. You can also count to three in your head. For example, "One Mississippi, two Mississippi, three Mississippi" will let 3 seconds pass. That's an easy thing to do in a situation that might get out of control. You count to three Mississippi in your mind, and chances are this will be enough time for the initial anger response to cool off.

> **Note to Therapists:** The effects of techniques such as visualizing a stop sign or counting to three alone have not been studied. However, as a 10-session package, this treatment is likely to be helpful. We hope that at least one of the techniques will resonate with a particular child and he will start using it on a daily basis. It is possible that some of these techniques may appear too simplistic to a child, and if this is the case, the therapist may just move on to the next section of the manual. Some children will have already heard about these approaches to anger management from their parents, teachers, or from previous therapy and may think that they do not work. The truth is that no one knows which one anger coping skill may be helpful in a particular situation and with a particular child. But by trying various coping skills over the course of a 10-week

program, the child may strengthen his emotion regulation and problem-solving skills, and with time these skills will become part of his second nature.

3.3. *Role-play the Stop & Think technique* using either situations reported by the child or hypothetical situations provided below. The therapist should read the provoking statement and the child must say "One Mississippi, two Mississippi, three Mississippi," and then say how he would have responded in this situation now that he's taken 3 seconds to cool off. During this role play, the therapist can model and provide enthusiastic praise for participation. Sample situations include:

Imagine you are at school and before class someone says, "Let me copy your homework. If you don't let me copy it, I'll tell the teacher that you copied yours."
Let's say you are playing basketball and one of the other kids says, "Get the hell out of here. You don't know how to play!"
At home your parent yells, "You can't watch TV! You have to do your homework and then clean your room!"

The therapist can use the **Stop Sign** handout as a prompt for the technique.

4. ***Discuss and practice using verbal reminders.*** Verbal reminders to relax and cool off when frustrated can help prevent escalations. Reminders are things that we say to ourselves to guide our behavior. Some people may sing or hum to themselves what they are doing to avoid forgetting important things—for example: "Put my keys in my pocket, da-da-da-na-na." Ask the child to name specific things he may do to remind himself to bring certain items to class.

4.1. *Give examples of reminders* (or self-instruction) used in pressure situations, such as what an athlete may say to himself before an important game. Ask the child to make a list of reminders that he might have used when playing sports or during tests. Some common examples are "Slow down," "Take it easy," "Take a deep breath," and "Concentrate."

4.2. *Practice using reminders.* It is best to use situations that have been previously brought up by the child. The therapist might say:

Imagine you are in a situation that you told me about before. You are watching TV and your sister turns the channel. Then when you take the remote, she pushes you. Of course, when your mother sees that you took the remote from your sister, you are sent to your room without TV. What reminders can you use when your sister turns the channel? How about when your mother tells you to go to your room? What can you say in your head when you are on your way to your room?

Have the child repeat one of the reminders, first out loud and then to himself. Provide praise for practicing and draw the difference between overt (audible) and covert (spoken to self) reminders. In our clinical experience we noticed that it might make it easier for children to remember using the reminders if they whisper a reminder rather than just think of it. In addition, whispering is an observable behavior, which allows for the parents to see or hear if the child is practicing this particular strategy.

4.3. *Relate the process of anger monitoring to the use of reminders.*

One other thing that you can remind yourself about is monitoring the intensity of your angry feelings. As a matter of fact, you can remind yourself to take your anger temperature before using the reminders. Just ask yourself a question: "How angry am I?" This can be a reminder to reflect on the intensity of your anger and then decide the best way to handle it.

For example, imagine you are sitting down for dinner and see that your mother reheated green beans and meatloaf from yesterday. She always insists that you eat your vegetables. You might think, "Green beans for dinner? Not again, I hate it!" This thought could be a cue to ask yourself a question: "Does this situation make me annoyed, angry, or furious?" Those three words stand for different levels of anger intensity. After considering this question, you might conclude that having green beans two days in a row is annoying but not infuriating and that you can tolerate the mild discomfort of chewing and swallowing the not-so-tasty food without getting into an argument with your mother about it.

5. ***Discuss verbal labels for angry feelings.*** The words that we use to label our emotional states may also affect the intensity of emotion. Verbal labels such as "I am so mad" can lead to increased arousal compared to "This is unpleasant." Briefly talk about synonyms for the word *anger* and explain how some synonyms indicate higher levels of anger intensity while others reflect milder levels of anger. Sometimes people automatically use inflammatory verbal labels to refer even to trivial situations. After they label an experience with a strong word or phrase ("I fu@*ing hate this sh%t"), they feel more emotionally aroused because of the inflammatory label.

5.1. *Expand the child's vocabulary for anger.* Use the **Words for Anger** handout to highlight the role that strong, inflammatory labels play in increasing the anger experience. For children who have a habit of using strong words, ask if there is a new word on the list that they like and might use instead. Practice using milder words such as "upset" or "disappointed" instead of stronger words such as "mad" and "pissed off," and suggest that the child tries to use milder words for anger at home.

5.2. *Model the inner talk that can be used to modify strong verbal labeling.*

Imagine that something annoying happened and you are very angry. You turn on your self-monitoring inner eye and check out the kind of thoughts that are going through your head. That's when you catch yourself thinking, "I am really pissed off!" There may be strong swear words also sounding in your head. That's when you remind yourself that when people use strong, inflammatory words, they get even angrier. Then you can say to yourself: "I am not pissed off, I am just frustrated."

Ask the child to provide two situations that would definitely make him angry and then practice using mild words for anger in response to these situations. These are some examples of hypothetical provocations:

You teacher failed you unfairly . . .   You can say to yourself . . .
Some guy called you a chicken . . .   You can say to yourself . . .

6.   ***Continue relaxation training.*** Ask if the child was able to use the deep breathing relaxation technique during the previous week. Relate the deep breathing technique to the Feeling Thermometer activity by asking the child to imagine how the red bar in the feeling thermometer goes down every time he exhales. The therapist may choose either to continue to practice the breathing technique or to introduce additional relaxation methods, some of which are described below. A rationale for using relaxation techniques can be given to the child in the following way:

Anger has a physiological component of arousal. "Physiological" refers to what your body feels when you are angry. For example, some people might feel the blood rushing to their face and their nostrils flaring when they are angry. These are the physiological signs of emotional arousal. Relaxation is the opposite of arousal. If you learn how to relax when you are starting to feel angry, you can prevent anger from building up.

6.1.   The *deep breathing and backward counting technique* was suggested by Eva Feindler (Feindler & Ecton, 1986). The therapist can first model the technique and then ask the child to practice while providing feedback. We found this technique to be particularly helpful to individuals who have clear signs of physiological anger arousal that last for up to several minutes.

Take a deep breath, and as you breathe out say the number 10 aloud. Take a deep breath, and as you breathe out say the number 9 aloud and then say, "I am more relaxed and calm at 9 than I was at 10." Take a deep breath, and as you breathe out say the number 8 and then say, "I am more relaxed and calm at 8 than I was at 9." Continue this procedure until you get to 1.

6.2.   Introduce the *deep breathing and pleasant thinking technique* by asking the child to close his eyes and use his imagination to describe a pleasant outdoor scene. Prompt him to be as descriptive as possible, asking about colors, sounds, and surroundings. This description could be 2 to 3 minutes in duration. After the description is detailed enough, ask the child to visualize himself in this pleasant situation and focus on slow, rhythmic breathing for a few minutes to achieve a state of calm relaxation.

Not everyone can hold on to the same mental image for several minutes, and children who don't seem to enjoy this technique may use a simpler relaxation method, such as taking a few deep breaths when they start to feel really angry.

7. ***Summarize the session and assign homework.*** Ask the child to recap the main points of the session and think of at least one way this material is relevant to the kinds of things that make him angry. The following script can be used to summarize Session 2:

> Today we spoke about monitoring our anger arousal. We spoke about different levels of anger intensity and about different words that we may use to name our feelings. Then we spoke about the Stop & Think technique. You have to stop for a few seconds and think about how you feel. If you feel angry, you can use the reminders to cool off. Finally, we did some relaxation practice. Which relaxation technique do you like the best?

7.1. Ask the child to *write down his favorite reminder on an index card and carry this card in his pocket for one day.* He should take it out and use it if there is a conflict or a provocation.

7.2. Ask the child to *practice all three of the relaxation techniques* (deep breathing, positive imagery, counting backward, and their combinations) several times over the course of the next week. The **Relaxation Practice Log 1** should be completed before the next session.

7.3. **Daily Anger Monitoring Logs** should be used only with motivated participants. Ask the child to record and briefly describe *all incidents* of anger that occur before the next session.

7.4. **Anger Management Log 2** should be filled out for the next session of the program. In this assignment, the child is asked to record only one episode in which he was able to effectively use one of the anger-control techniques practiced in the previous session. This assignment should enhance the generalization of anger management skills to real-life circumstances.

8. ***Check in with parent(s).*** At the end of each session, parent(s) or guardian(s) can be invited for a brief check-in to review material of the session, progress during the past week, and the anger management plan for the next week. We find it best to have these family meetings focus on the positive behaviors such as the child's ability to navigate frustrating situations without an anger outburst. If particular incidents of disruptive behavior need to be discussed, it is advisable to ask the child to wait outside and have this discussion one-on-one with the parent.

Ask the parents to give an example of a situation in which their child was able to engage in appropriate behavior (e.g., walked away from a fight, took out the trash when asked only once) in a situation that could have triggered anger or noncompliance. Ask the child to tell his parents what he learned in session. If needed, therapists may provide two or three bullet points from the session material that resonated most with the child.

Emotion Regulation

 GOALS

1. Collect homework and review the previous session's material.
2. Review progress to date.
3. Discuss ways to prevent anger-provoking situations.
4. Discuss the monitoring of anger cues.
5. Continue relaxation training: progressive muscle relaxation.
6. Summarize the session and assign homework.
7. Check in with parent(s).

 HANDOUTS

Feeling Thermometer

Where Do You Feel Anger Inside?

The Many Faces of Anger

Drawing Anger

✓ **HOMEWORK**

Progressive Muscle Relaxation (optional)

Anger Management Log 3

Relaxation Practice Log 2

Creative activity (optional, no handout)

1.   ***Collect homework and review the previous session's material.*** If the child brings in the completed homework, provide appropriate praise and briefly discuss any reported anger-provoking situations. If the child has not done the homework, gently stress the importance of filling out the forms at home. Take a few minutes to ask about anger episodes during the past week.

1.1.   Briefly review the last session's material and *ask for examples of times the child was able to use the Stop & Think technique, verbal reminders, and relaxation techniques.*

The goal of this program is to reduce unpleasant anger. So far, we've discussed some of the situations that make people angry, and we've spoken about several strategies for improving one's bad mood. Today I would like to talk more about the intensity of anger. Remember how last time we spoke about the Feeling Thermometer? I'd like for you to learn to keep your anger temperature at the cool level, so that you don't have these episodes of rage and extreme anger when your emotions seem to go through the roof. Last time we discussed using reminders and relaxation techniques as ways to regulate anger arousal.

1.2.   *Review Anger Management Log 2* and praise successful attempts to use anger control techniques. If the child does not bring any written accounts, fill out the Anger Management Log together so that it can be used as an example during this session.

2.   ***Review progress to date.***

> **Note to Therapists:** The key to a flexible implementation of this manualized treatment is continuing to monitor the child's progress and motivation. The best-case scenario is that after the second session the child will have some success with anger management and the parents will also report a reduction in the number and intensity of anger outbursts and aggressive behavior. This initial success, in turn, will strengthen cooperation for the remainder of the treatment.
>
> It is also possible that children who are referred for disruptive behavior at home and/or at school may also have a negative attitude about being in therapy. This may manifest itself in lack of interest and resistance to activities in session and failure to produce written homework. When asked directly, some of the more honest participants have told us after the first few sessions that the anger-control program is "useless." These comments are best countered by being open about the effectiveness of behavioral therapy. The therapist can say that it usually helps a little over half of people who try it, but stress that it is important to finish the full program in order to know whether it works or not. Remarkably, by the end of the 10th session, most children, even those who did not show improvement on the outcome measures, had something positive to say about this treatment.

Therapists should do their best to be engaging; this may include taking on topics of interest to children such as video games, sports, and music. However, there is a fine line between being entertaining and covering the material of the treatment manual. It takes a certain familiarity with the manual to be able to weave rapport-building efforts into the goals of the treatment. For example, we have asked children to draw a picture of the problem situation to make the discussion a bit livelier. On several occasions we have encouraged the children to show us their favorite game on an iPod or a portable game player at the end of a session in order to finish the session on a positive note. There are also examples of more structured reward systems. For example, tokens awarded for each 10 minutes of active participation could then be exchanged for small prizes at the end of the session, but we have not used this method in our work. We have found that the best way to deal with resistance is by providing enthusiastic delivery of the material and consistent but gentle encouragement to participate in the activities outlined in the handouts. In our clinical experience, children who made us work the hardest to win their interest were also the ones who made the most use of the emotion regulation and problem-solving skills after they get on board with the program.

2.1. *Ask the child for feedback about the program to date.*

> Well, it has been 2 weeks, and I would like to see if we are moving in the right direction. Do you think the first two sessions we've had have been beneficial to you in any way?

In our experience, most children can say something positive about the program after the first two sessions. If a child can name something that has been beneficial, the therapist can elicit further information or a specific example that describes how he benefited. If a child says nothing has been beneficial so far, the therapist can note that the child is still in the very early part of treatment and that hopefully future sessions will be more helpful.

2.2. It is always useful *to reiterate the goals of the program* in a way that shows how the program can benefit the child.

> If you don't spend all this time arguing with your mom, you can have more time to play.
> If you use your words next time your sister gives you a hard time, you won't be grounded.

3. **Discuss ways to prevent anger-provoking situations.** One of the most effective ways to reduce anger is by preventing anger-provoking situations in the first place. Of course, this strategy won't work every time. Some anger-provoking situations are unavoidable, and those have to be confronted and resolved. When this is the case, it's important to remember that while it's OK to be mad, it's not OK to be mean. Another point is that people with anger control problems (high trait anger, low frustration tolerance, etc.) can be angered by the most trivial and benign situations. However, learning to recognize potential provocations and learning to distinguish the important from the inconsequential ones is a helpful anger control skill. The goal of this section is to expand the child's awareness of events that may trigger his anger.

Discuss whether events that make the child angry can be prevented or ignored. If the child has completed the weekly **Anger Monitoring Logs** as part of his homework from the first two sessions, the therapists can use anger-triggering events reported in the logs. Alternatively, the therapist may use examples of anger episodes reported during the sessions.

Use the definitions from the list below and ask the child to describe the difference between avoidable versus unavoidable situations and situations that can be ignored versus situations that cannot be ignored.

> Avoidable = can be prevented.
> Unavoidable = cannot be prevented.
> Can be ignored = not worth being upset about.
> Cannot be ignored = something has to be done.

Our first strategy is prevention. Let's look at some of the situations when you got angry or frustrated over the past 2 weeks. You described several times when [fill in with an example from the child's homework]. Let's sort these situations into two groups, those that can be prevented and those that cannot be prevented. What could be done to prevent these situations from occurring? For those that could not be prevented, what are some ways you could have managed your anger in order to end up with the best possible outcome?

3.1. *Prompt the child to generate a few strategies for preventing situations that are likely to make him angry.* It is not uncommon for children to know the right answer even if they seldom perform the behavior. After offering several prevention strategies, ask the child to estimate the chances that he will actually use the strategy. The therapist can either use a simple scale—such as definitely, maybe, probably not—or record the child's own words. This prediction can be used as a comparison to actual behavior during the next session.

These are some possible examples of prevention strategies that were offered by participants of this program: "Think ahead," "Don't go there," "Tell people that you might get angry," "Give them a warning," "Take a time-out," "Leave the room," "Drink a glass of water."

3.2. An alternative approach is to *build a hierarchy of anger-provoking situations.* Situations can be grouped into categories based on the levels of anger intensity. Then, different levels of anger intensity can be matched to various anger management techniques. The goal of this exercise is to improve the child's ability to predict his level of anger and to match an emotion regulation technique to the levels of anger.

4.   ***Discuss the monitoring of anger cues.*** Paradoxically, individuals who are prone to high levels of anger are very sensitive to external anger cues (provocation), but may be unaware of internal cues (such as the intensity of emotional arousal, physiological changes, and levels of stress, fatigue, or hunger that may predispose a person to overreact). Consequently, it is helpful to work on self-monitoring skills that can be used to detect the early signs of what may become an explosive anger outburst. This message could be communicated to children as follows:

> If you recall our firecracker picture, people may have a very short fuse for certain triggers of anger. Or, to use another analogy, a sports car can blast to 60 miles per hour in less than 5 seconds. You see, the goal of this program is to slow down your emotional reaction time so that you don't accelerate so fast. [The **Feeling Thermometer** introduced in the previous session can be used as a visual aid.] Right now, you go from discomfort to rage almost instantly. I want you to go first from unpleasant to uncomfortable, then from uncomfortable to annoyed, then from annoyed to frustrated, and so on. This way, you go through several levels of intensity before you might get to the top. If you can also monitor these increments in terms of the intensity of your anger, then when you notice that the intensity of your anger is rising, you can use prevention strategies to prevent an explosive outburst. In other words, anger is not an all-or-nothing reaction. It has several levels of intensity, and if you monitor the intensity of emotional arousal, you can use different strategies to prevent explosions.

4.1.   *Review physiological cues.*

> Let's talk about how anger feels inside. What happens to our body when we are angry? Where is anger located?

To make this discussion a little more engaging, therapists can use the **Where Do You Feel Anger Inside?** handout, which features an outline of a person, and ask the child to draw where it feels to be angry. Some of the common responses to the question "What happens to our body when we are angry?" include "My heart pounds," "My muscles tense up," "Blood rushes through my body," "My ears burn," "I frown," "My fists clench," "There are butterflies in my stomach," "My body shakes." Use this activity to help children identify cues of tension and point out that these are the cues that can be addressed by relaxation.

4.2.   *Review facial expressions of anger.*

> What do people look like when they are angry?

A good way to introduce this topic is to ask the child to make an angry face, then a happy face, a sad face, a surprised face, and a scared face. Then the therapist can also make angry, happy, and sad faces and ask the child to identify the emotions. Anger and happiness are the easiest to recognize, and if done correctly, this exercise usually brings some comic relief to the session. Interestingly, while most of us look angry when we feel angry, sometimes looking angry can actually *cause* us to feel angry. In a psychological experiment some people were asked to bite on a pencil while others were not, and all were asked to rate how they would feel in a variety of anger-provoking situations. Those who had their teeth clenched (by biting on a pencil) reported being more angry. Use **The Many Faces of Anger** handout and ask the child to describe how he looks when he is angry.

4.3.   A *creative activity* can be useful, especially with younger children, in producing a description of internal experiences of anger. One of the possible reasons that some children express their anger inappropriately is because they may not have sufficient vocabulary to explain how they feel. An engaging way to expand children's awareness of anger experiences and enhance the potential for appropriate verbal expression of that anger is to ask the child to draw a picture showing how anger feels to him (use the **Drawing Anger** handout). Explain that this picture does not have to look like anything he has ever seen. To help the child get started, ask him to remember a time when he was really mad and to recall how he felt at that moment. The drawing can be discussed using the following opening questions:

What colors best show how you feel when you get mad?
How would you make an angry shape?

5.   ***Continue relaxation training: Progressive muscle relaxation.*** Children who have responded well to the deep breathing and positive imagery techniques in the previous session can be introduced to progressive muscle relaxation. In our experience with muscle relaxation, it is only helpful if practiced every day over the course of at least several weeks. Most children who participated in this program with us opted out of doing progressive muscle relaxation exercises every day. However, a small minority found it to be helpful. Hence, we suggest that therapists introduce this technique to everyone but only keep it as an ongoing technique for those who are really motivated to use it on a consistent basis. It is also useful to conduct progressive muscle relaxation training at least once during this session to provide an experiential example of the difference between feelings of tension and relaxation. This may help children be better able to identify their states of excessive tension. Provide the following rationale:

By physically tensing your muscles and then relaxing them, you will be able to recognize the difference between feeling tense and feeling relaxed. I will ask you to sit in a comfortable position and close your eyes. Then I will tell you to tense and then relax different muscle groups. Upon tensing, breathe in through your nose and count to 5. Then when I say "now relax," breathe out through your mouth, releasing the tension in that muscle group, and feel the difference between tension and relaxation. For example, I want you to make a tight fist. Now count to 5. Now open your fingers and rest your palm on your lap for 10 seconds. Do you feel the difference between tension and relaxation in your hand? Wait 10 seconds, paying close attention to the relaxed feeling in that particular muscle group (such as warmth, heaviness, looseness, and tingling sensation in the muscles). Now let's do this exercise for all the main muscle groups.

Therapists can also model the movements that are used to relax the major muscle groups. The sequence below has been adapted from Edmund Jacobson's original relaxation exercises. It is recommended that each muscle group be tensed and relaxed twice. Hold tension for at least 5 seconds and then relax for at least 10 seconds. Concentrate on breathing in through the nose and out through the mouth.

Abbreviated Sequence for Muscle Relaxation
1. Clench both fists → hands and forearms
2. Bend both elbows → biceps
3. Frown and clench teeth → face and jaw
4. Push head back and down → neck
5. Push shoulder blades together → shoulders and back
6. Tense stomach muscles → abdominal region
7. Raise legs out, curling feet → thighs
8. Keep legs up, curl toes down → calves, feet, and toes.

6. *Summarize the session and assign homework.* Ask the child to summarize what he has learned in the session. The following summary can also be provided:

Today we spoke about the intensity of anger and about emotional arousal that we experience when we are angry. We spoke about how to monitor the levels of emotional arousal, which go from low to high. Then we discussed different cues, such as how our body reacts to stress and facial expressions. The take-home message is that it is important to know about the level of our anger so that we can prevent bad things that might happen if the anger explodes.

6.1. If the child has been completing the **Daily Anger Monitoring Log** and it has been helpful in sessions, you can continue this assignment. However, therapists may decide to discontinue this form to avoid excessive burden and allow the child to focus on practicing other anger management strategies. The daily log can be used again at Sessions 8 and 9 in order to collect information about the number of anger episodes during the last 2 weeks of the program.

6.2. It is important that the child has opportunities to *practice relaxation techniques at home.* Children who responded well to the progressive muscle relaxation in session can be given the **Progressive Muscle Relaxation** handout to practice at home. Use the **Relaxation Practice Log 2** to record the day, time, and location of all attempts to use rhythmic breathing, positive imagery, counting backward, and muscle relaxation.

6.3. **Anger Management Log 3** should be filled out for the next session of the program. In this assignment, the child is asked to record one episode each week in which he effectively used one of the anger control techniques. Because this session focused on prevention and self-monitoring of anger arousal, encourage the child to pick an instance for this week's assignment in which he used these specific skills.

6.4. An *optional creative assignment* can be given. In the creative spirit of this session, children can be asked to write a one-page essay about an anger episode that occurs before the next session. Some participants of this program have produced amazingly astute works of writing. We also received creative projects in the format of Power-Point presentations, computer-generated cartoon animations, and videos. These assignments are hard to manualize, but we encourage therapists to add creative elements.

7. ***Check in with parent(s).*** At the end of each session, parent(s) or guardian(s) can be invited for a brief check-in to review material of the session, progress during the past week, and the anger management plan for the next week. Ask the parent to give an example of a time when their child was able to engage in appropriate behavior (e.g., walked away from a fight, took out the trash when asked only once) in a situation that could have triggered anger or noncompliance. Ask the child to tell his parents what he learned in session. If needed, therapists may provide two or three bullet points from the session material that resonated most with the child.

MODULE 2

PROBLEM SOLVING

Problem Identification and Attribution

GOALS

1. Collect homework and review the previous session's material.
2. Discuss the connection between thoughts and emotions.
3. Introduce problem identification.
4. Discuss perspective taking.
5. Discuss hostile attribution bias.
6. Summarize the session and assign homework.
7. Check in with parent(s).

MATERIALS

Pictures from magazines or books (see Section 5.2)

HANDOUTS

Calming Thoughts
Blind Men and a Large Object

HOMEWORK

Anger Management Log 4

1. ***Collect homework and review the previous session's material.*** Ask the child to recall the contents of the previous session. Review **Anger Management Log 3** and discuss self-monitoring for anger arousal cues to prevent uncontrollable anger outbursts. Ask for at least one example when the child was able to recognize that he was getting angry and was able to use this awareness to prevent further escalation of anger.

1.1. *Inquire about whether the child has been using relaxation techniques at home.*

Technique	Has the child used this at home?		Did he find it useful?	
Rhythmic breathing	Yes	No	Yes	No
Positive imagery	Yes	No	Yes	No
Counting backward	Yes	No	Yes	No
Muscle relaxation	Yes	No	Yes	No

So far, we have been talking about anger as a feeling. We've also discussed different situations that make people angry and different anger management skills. In the next few sessions, we will talk about how our thinking can be related to our emotions. As Shakespeare wrote: "There is nothing either good or bad, but thinking makes it so."

Note to Therapists: There are multiple theories of the role of cognition in anger and aggression. Sessions 4–6 of this protocol utilize the social information-processing model, which has resulted in hundreds of studies on aggression and disruptive behavior in children (Crick & Dodge, 1994; Dodge, 2006). This model suggests that there are five steps in cognitive processing of social information: detection of cues, interpretation of cues, solution generation, analysis of consequences, and response enactment. At all steps, there could be two types of problems, cognitive deficits (not engaging a particular process) and cognitive deficiencies (making an error in processing), that are related to anger and aggressive behavior. Several social problem–solving interventions that aim to correct these cognitive problems vary in terms of relative complexity and emphasis on one process over the other (Guerra & Slaby, 1990; Kazdin et al., 1987; Lochman et al., 2008; Shure & Spivack, 1982). A common theme of these approaches is using cognitive restructuring techniques to target constructs implicated in aggressive behavior including beliefs supporting aggression, hostile attribution bias, and lack of insight into the motives of other people.

Similarly, cognitive processes such as inflammatory labeling, misattribution of intent, and blaming are involved in the experience of the emotion of anger. Indeed, cognitive reappraisal has been one of the earliest techniques for dealing with excessive anger within the framework of rational-emotive therapy (Ellis, 1977).

2. ***Discuss the connection between thoughts and emotions.*** This topic can be introduced to children in the following way:

There are different ways in which anger and thinking can be connected. For example, a person can get angry because of a misunderstanding. We have discussed how acting without thinking can get people in trouble. Remember how you told me [give an example relevant to this client]? Sometimes we can make mistakes in our thinking and get angry as a consequence of these mistakes. For example, you might think that your friend broke your cell phone, but in fact he never even touched it. In other words, we can get angry because we misunderstood something. Can you remember a time when someone got angry at you because of a misunderstanding—for example, a time when your parents might have thought you did something that you did not do?

2.1. *Remembering old grudges can make a person angry.* A therapist might ask a child to recall something that made him really angry and describe that situation for a few moments.

For example, you told me about [recall one of the high-anger situations that was previously discussed in session]. Let's do a little experiment. I will ask you to think back to this event and recall it in as much detail as you can. Take a few seconds to remember and reflect on how angry you were back then.

Wait for a few seconds while the child thinks back, and then ask if thinking about something that made him angry in the past can still make him angry now.

2.2. On the one hand, acting without thinking can cause problems. On the other hand, *thinking too much or being unable to let go of thoughts about anger-provoking events may lead to excessive anger.* A construct of anger rumination is a helpful way to capture various maladaptive thought processes associated with the emotion of anger (Sukhodolsky, Golub, & Cromwell, 2001). A simple way to educate children about the effect of their thinking on their anger is to distinguish between "hot, cool, and calming" thoughts. Hot thoughts make us angrier. This topic can be considered as an extension of the "reminders" and verbal labeling techniques from the previous session, except that instead of using one phrase or one word, the child is guided to monitor his inner monologue and to use calming self-talk instead of letting automatic and likely inflammatory thoughts pop up in their heads.

Often when we are angry, we have inflammatory thoughts in our head. For example, if your mom tells you that you have to turn off your computer and start your homework, you may think, "She always does this to me" or "It's unfair." You may have the same thought every time you run into a problem with your mom. Or you may think, "He is so stupid, I'm gonna kill him for that," when your friend does something that makes you angry. These are examples of hot thoughts—thoughts that may make us angrier.

We can use our inner voice to talk ourselves out of being angry. We have already practiced some simple things that we can say in our head to stop being angry. Do you remember what I am talking about? When you say things such as "relax," "cool off," and so on, we call these phrases "Reminders."

Children are asked to make a list of three things that make them angry and then make a list of what they could think about in each of these situations in order to calm down. Ask the child to fill out the **Calming Thoughts** handout and lead the discussion on how thoughts can be related to anger. Ask the child to give his own definition of hot thoughts, cool thoughts, and calming thoughts. For example, one child in our program reported that a kid in his music class was throwing paperclips at him when the teacher was not looking, and he made a list of thoughts that went through his mind:

I'm gonna punch him in the face.
Human nature is driving me crazy.
It's not worth getting all worked up about.
He is an idiot; I don't need to stoop to his level.

In this example, thinking the first two thoughts are likely to make a person angrier and thinking the third and fourth thoughts is likely to make a person less angry, although the choice of words to characterize the instigator in the first clause of the fourth example could have been better.

3.   ***Introduce problem identification.*** The first step of problem solving is identifying something as a problem. Anger acts as an important signal that something is a problem and gives us energy to find a solution. For example, a politician can be driven by anger at the injustices of the world. Of course, being angry or frustrated can reduce our ability to problem-solve if we make less-than-optimal choices or fail to understand the perspectives of the other people involved in the situation. Our goals are also integral components of problem identification, and circumstances that thwart our goals are perceived as problems.

Let's talk about how we know there is a problem. A problem exists when something gets in the way of a goal we want to reach or keeps us from getting what we want. A problem can also exist if two people want different goals and both goals cannot be met with one simple solution. People can sometimes tell when there is a problem because they feel angry or sad.

For example, one girl who participated in this program was getting mad at her mother when she was doing something on her computer and her mother was telling her to get off. The problem was that this girl was usually doing something that required time to finish, such as updating her iPod play list, and her mom's request interrupted the project. Of course, this girl's mother wanted her daughter to get to the dinner table while the food was still warm. Can you think what was the problem in this situation for the girl and what was the problem for her mother?

3.1.   As an example of problem identification, *ask the child to imagine that his video game system is not working.*

Can you think of what can possibly be wrong?

You can mention different observations and ask the child to suggest what those might indicate about the problem. For example:

Observation	Potential problem
The light is not on.	Not plugged in
The picture comes on but the figures don't move.	Controls not working
The TV screen is on but the game doesn't appear.	No disc
The TV works, but nothing happens when you turn on the game.	Broken processor

Ask the child to offer information that would help to identify the problem.

3.2. *Now introduce another person to the problem situation.*

Now imagine that your brother broke the system; how would this change the situation? What would be your goals: To have the system fixed? To get your brother punished?

Problems that involve other people are, obviously, much more likely to lead to conflicts and arguments. Being able to understand when there is a problem is the first step toward controlling your reactions and getting along.

Usually when there is a problem, our initial reaction is to try and get what we want. But there are other goals too, such as to stay out of trouble, having friends who like you, and getting along with your brother even though he might have broken the video game.

4. *Discuss perspective taking.* The purpose of this section is to help children understand different points of view. Different people can perceive the same problem from different angles, and consequently their understanding of what the problem is may be different. One way to explain this point is through the consideration of goals. For instance, people perceive problems differently because they have different goals when they interact with each other. For example:

When Ginny came home after school, she wanted to go play soccer with her friends. However, before she could leave the house, her mother stopped her and said that she could only go outside after she finished her homework. She reminded her that she has not been doing well in school, and one way to change that is to be sure she always completes her homework.

Ask the child to define the problem in the situation. If the child suggests that the problem is that her mom is not fair or that Ginny never gets to do what she wants, discuss how this problem definition may actually hinder problem solving, because there is little that the child can do to resolve the problem since she cannot control her mother's actions. The therapist can ask questions such as:

What is the problem according to the mom?
What is the problem according to Ginny?

How did this problem start?
What is Ginny's goal?
What is the mother's goal?
Knowing the mother's goal, what can Ginny do so that she won't get in trouble?

4.1. *Ask the child to describe how situations can be perceived differently by the different people who are involved in them.* Here are examples of some situations that can be used:

Your friend steps on your toes and keeps walking.
You sit in gum on the school bus and the kid next to you starts laughing.
You trip over your friend's foot while playing outside.

Alternatively, take some of the problem situations reported by the child earlier and reexamine how these situations could have been seen by the other people involved.

4.2. Use the **Blind Men and a Large Object** exercise to further illustrate how people may have different perceptions of the same situation. This activity can be particularly useful with younger children or with children who are more reserved during the session.

Let me tell you a story about a group of blind men who came across a large object and were trying to figure out what it was. They felt it with their hands and each came up with a different opinion:

"What I feel is like a fan."
"What I feel is like a tree."
"What I feel is like a rope."
"What I feel is like a horn."
"What I feel is like a high wall."
"What I feel is like a snake."

In reality, they were all right. The "object" was actually an elephant. Can you think of ways in which different parts of an elephant are like all of these different things?

An alternative way to present this activity is to tell the child the descriptions of different parts of the same object that the blind men were touching and to ask him to guess what it is. With younger children, a therapist can ask the child to draw each descriptive piece on the **Blind Men and a Large Object** handout. After all parts are drawn, see if they can fit together as one object.

Sometimes we only have information about part of the situation. We can easily make mistakes in judging what's going on when we don't have all the information. We can best understand the problem when we consider what other people saw or what they think about the situation.

5.   *Discuss hostile attribution bias.* The hostile attribution bias is one of the common social-cognitive distortions that may lead to excessive anger and aggression. It refers to thinking that another person is responsible for some negative outcome. Use situations reported by the child in the **Anger Management Logs** or throughout the sessions to explore the topic of causality: Why did the situation happen? Who was responsible? Was it an accident or did someone do it on purpose? If a child reveals a consistent belief that bad situations are caused by other people acting on purpose, it could be a sign of hostile attribution bias.

    Consider the following examples:

He did it because he hates me (teacher).
He did it because he is an idiot (peer).
She always does this to me (mother).

Guide the child to come up with alternative explanations. For example:

He did it because he had a headache.
He did it because he was not looking.
She did it because she was stressed out after coming home from work.

It is important to understand what the other person is thinking before we act in response. When we get into arguments with other people, it is often because we don't know what they really want or think. We get the wrong idea about where they're coming from. This usually happens because, without thinking, we quickly come to believe that the other person wanted to hurt us or do something bad to us on purpose. Most of the time, though, there is another reason for this person's behavior. This is why we have to try and understand what motivates the other person's actions.

5.1.   One goal of this section is to *identify the intentions and goals of other people.* First, the therapist may present four simple categories of people's intention or motives. The list is not exhaustive, and it can be modified to match the child's age and level of social sophistication. The following four motives can be written down on a white board or piece of paper.

> 1. **Being helpful**: good intention—"They are trying to help me out."
> 2. **Being mean**: hostile intention—"They were trying to make me angry or upset."
> 3. **Don't know**: unclear intention—"It is unclear why they did that."
> 4. **Accidental**: unintentional behavior—"They accidentally did what they did."

Then the therapist should read the two ambiguous vignettes below and ask the child to identify the character's intention from the list of motives just reviewed.

    1. Imagine that you are getting lunch in the school cafeteria. You have your lunch on the tray and when you are walking back to your table, you slip on something. As you are trying to keep your balance, your tray starts to wobble and the food is about to slide

down on the floor. Someone reaches over to grab the tray but instead of catching it he knocks your drink all over your clothes.

2. Imagine that you are working on your homework and have about half of your report typed up when your mother calls you for dinner. You go right away because you are very hungry, and you forget to save your file. Everyone sits down for a nice dinner. After dinner is over, you have to call a friend to ask her something. At that time your brother goes on the computer to play his game, and he closes your homework file without saving it.

Discuss how it is unclear from the stories if it was an accident or if the other child caused the problem on purpose.

5.2. A *creative exercise* can be helpful in prompting the child to think about other peoples' motives. The therapist can create a file of pictures from magazines or books that show groups of people interacting. Some pictures should show people looking happy, sad, or angry. Some pictures should show people participating in physical activities like skiing or playing soccer while others should show people simply conversing in various contexts. For example, a picture of schoolchildren working on a project could be used with a child who might have incidents of disruptive behavior in school. A picture of an adult talking to a child could be used with a child whose targeted behavioral problems include noncompliance. The therapist can either ask questions about the picture or instruct the child to write a short story using the questions as guidelines.

Can you make up a story about what is going on in this picture? Who is the main character? What does he want? What is he thinking? Who are the other people? What do they want? What are they thinking?

As the child describes the actions and intentions of the characters, the therapist can write them down. Ask the child how he might respond if approached by a person with the intentions he identifies in the picture. The activity can be concluded by discussing the list of intentions generated by the child and highlighting how people in one situation may have different goals. The child's responses can be rephrased to map on the categories of motives from the previous exercise involving the vignettes of the session (helpful or mean, unclear or accidental).

Throughout the exercise, the therapist should emphasize that it is often difficult to know why someone did something. Encourage the child to remind himself not to jump to conclusions about the other person's intentions, and to consider different possible explanations for other people's actions.

We should be careful when thinking about the intentions of other people. What we think about the other person's motivation may influence our reaction toward this person. To avoid jumping to conclusions that might be wrong, and which might lead to a conflict, consider different reasons for people's behavior.

5.3. Discuss how *being angry can lead us to ignore cues that someone may be trying to be helpful*. For example, being frustrated with the lost homework project in the earlier vignette, a child might think that the mother who asked "What happened?" is trying to blame him rather than help. Being extremely frustrated may create a "blind spot" in our ability to clearly see other people's intentions.

Sometimes we forget to think about other explanations for why bad things happen because anger can cause us to have "blind spots." Blind spots happen when we let feelings from past situations affect how we see other people in situations that are happening now. Similarly, teachers might have blind spots that affect how they see you and your behavior in the classroom. Parents may have a blind spot when they still think about an old conflict and interpret current events in terms of an old situation. Can you think of any blind spots that you may have when you are angry or frustrated?

6. *Summarize the session and assign homework.* Ask the child to summarize what he has learned in the session. Therapists can also conclude the session contents by paraphrasing some of the client's relevant comments.

Today we discussed the connection between thinking and anger. We talked about how hot and cool thoughts can change the intensity of anger. Then we spoke about problem identification. Sometimes if we stop to think and ask ourselves "Is there a problem?", we realize that actually there is no problem and there is nothing to be angry about. For example, if you thought your brother turned off the computer without saving your homework project, you might get angry for only a moment before you realize you'd saved the project in a different folder than you originally thought.

Next we said that problems happen when we don't get what we want or when our goals are not met. We outlined some goals that we can set for ourselves in order to better deal with conflict situations. Then we spoke about how to understand the other person's goals and intentions. What we do, and whether we react with anger, may depend on what we think about this person's intentions toward us.

6.1. **Anger Management Log 4** should be filled out for the next session of the program. The child should record one episode during the week when he was able to effectively observe the motivation of another person in a conflict situation.

7. *Check in with parent(s).* At the end of each session, parent(s) or guardian(s) can be invited for a brief check-in to review material of the session, progress during the past week, and the anger management plan for the next week. Ask the parent to give an example of a time when their child was able to engage in appropriate behavior (e.g., walked away from a fight, took out the trash when asked only once) in a situation that could have triggered anger or noncompliance. Ask the child to tell his parents what he learned in session. If needed, therapists may provide two or three bullet points from the session material that resonated most with the child.

Generating Solutions

 ## GOALS

1. Collect homework and review the previous session's material.
2. Introduce the PICC handout.
3. Practice generating a range of solutions to problem situations.
4. Discuss the effects of anger on problem-solving ability.
5. Reinforce the use of appropriate verbal solutions.
6. Summarize the session and assign homework.
7. Check in with parent(s).

 ## HANDOUTS

Problem Identification, Choices, and Consequences (PICC)

Manage Anger before Problem Solving (MAPS)

Words to Express Anger Politely

☑ HOMEWORK

Anger Management Log 5

PICC (optional)

MAPS (optional)

1. **_Collect homework and review the previous session's material._** Ask the child to recall the contents of the previous session. If needed, summarize the last session by saying:

> Last time we spoke about problem identification. Did you have a chance to use this knowledge during the past week? We also spoke about different goals that people might have in a conflict situation. Did you have a chance to think about other people's goals using what we discussed last time? We also spoke about people's intentions; why do people do what they do?

1.1. *Review the situation reported in Anger Management Log 4* and emphasize that there are different ways to understand other people's behaviors and intentions. If needed, go over some of the categories of intentions, as presented in the previous session.

1.2. If the child brought in any *additional, overdue, or creative assignments*, review them and encourage practice of anger management skills between sessions.

2. **_Introduce the PICC handout._** This chart integrates the key steps of the social problem–solving model (Lochman et al., 2008). Problem identification refers to thinking about anger-provoking situations and conflicts in terms of one's own goals as well as the goals and motives of other people involved. Being able to generate multiple solutions (choices) and anticipate the outcomes (consequences) for each of the possible solutions are the social-problem skills needed for preventing or resolving conflicts. The following script can be used to introduce this topic.

> Every time we do something, there is a mental plan of action. We may not be aware of it, it might be unconscious, but every time we do something, there is a mental program that regulates our behavior. This mental program is not unlike computer software. When we learn to do something new, it's like downloading new software. For example, think about learning to ride a bike: at first it's hard and you fall, but once you know how to do it, riding a bike becomes second nature, you never forget how to do it. By the same token, when you have a problem to solve, there can be a mental plan helping you decide what you say and do. Today we'll talk about a blueprint for building an effective problem-solving strategy. If you practice it long enough, it will become as natural as riding a bike, so that you will automatically do the best possible thing when there is a problem you have to handle.

2.1. Use the **Problem Identification, Choices, and Consequences (PICC)** handout to aid discussion about each step of successful problem solving.

> We will use this PICC chart to "pick apart" problems and to "pick" good choices that really work for you.

Here is an example of a completed PICC chart:

I. *Problem Identification*

   1. What was the problem? *My sister switched the channel when I was watching TV.*

   2. What did you do? *Hit her with a pillow.*

   3. What did the other person do? *She told mom and I had to go to my room and could not finish watching my show.*

II. *Choices*   III. *Consequences* (for each choice)

   A. What could you have been done in the situation?

      1. I could have *punched her*   1. *more trouble for me*

      2. I could have *told her my show would be over soon*   2. *she wouldn't care*

      3. I could have *watched my show on an old TV*   3. *then she'd always watch big screen TV in the other room*

   B. What is the best choice (solution) to this problem? *I could have told her that my show would be over in 5 minutes and then she could watch whatever she wants.*

---

3.   ***Practice generating a range of solutions to problem situations.*** The purpose of this section is to assist children with better understanding the nature of problem solving, as well as to become better able to identify different possible solutions for problem situations. The therapist can use one of the problems previously reported by the child and have him generate as many solutions as possible.

I want you to tell me as many solutions to this problem as you can think of, no matter how silly you think it is.

As the child names various solutions, the therapist should write them down in a summary form. Then the solutions can be classified in some categories. For example:

Help seeking: asking someone to help you, telling the teacher.
Negotiation: asking for or telling what you want, trying to settle the problem.
Verbal aggression: saying something mean, being sarcastic.
Physical aggression: fighting, hitting.
Avoidance: avoiding the problem but in a way that it may come back later.

3.1.   If the child has difficulty generating solutions to real-life situations, *use a hypothetical story.* You can add a competitive edge by saying that there are eight possible solutions (listed below), and that you want to see how many of them the child can generate in 2 minutes.

Let's take a hypothetical situation. Imagine you are texting your friend after school and another boy comes by and grabs your phone away from you. He then starts to look at the pictures that you have stored on your phone. What are all the possible ways that you could solve this problem?

Possible Solutions
1. Forget about the phone for now, he will give it back later.
2. Demand that the boy give the phone back.
3. Tell the boy that you were in the middle of sending an important message.
4. Go tell a teacher.
5. Try to grab the phone back.
6. Go find an adult to help you get the phone back.
7. Go sit on the bench by yourself.
8. Find your friends and tell them.

Place the solutions in the categories, either the same as above, or in categories that would seem more appropriate for the client. This type of categorization helps to develop a cognitive schema for how problems can be solved. Lead the discussion to a conclusion that the best choices lead to the consequences that solve the problems and allow us to maintain friendships and avoid trouble.

3.2. *Practice problem solving with peers, parents, and teachers.*

Now let's try to fill out another **PICC** handout for a problem that you had with a teacher (then with a parent, then with a peer).

Role-play the best-choice solution for each of the three situations. The therapist may use the role-reversal technique, asking the child to take on the role of the other person while the therapist takes on the role of the child. After that, the therapist can switch back and have the child role-play himself while the therapist role-plays the other person.

4. **Discuss the effects of anger on problem-solving ability.** Negative emotions can interfere with thinking in general and with thinking about social situations in particular. The therapist can relate the problem-solving information to the material from the first four sessions and guide the discussion by using the following points:

The feeling of anger can stir up hostile thoughts.
Anger can drive us to act before we have time to think about a good plan of action.
Anger can reduce our ability to calmly talk about the problem.

Use one of the previously filled out **Anger Management Logs** to discuss a solution to a real-life problem that was described by the child. Ask whether being angry at that moment had an effect on his ability to generate solutions. The effect of anger on problem solving may be compared to having a blind spot or tunnel vision.

When we are angry, our ability to understand the problem or to think about our choices may narrow. We only see what's in front of us, and can't see anything on the sides, like when we are driving in a tunnel. The goal is to get out of the tunnel and see what's around us. So, when we talk about different solutions here in the clinic, it looks like you have no problem coming up with a great number of different choices. The trick is to be able to use those problem-solving skills when some conflict actually happens to you in real life.

4.1.　*Link anger monitoring and other emotion regulation techniques with problem-solving skills.* Ask the child to use the clearest cue that he may be angry (situational, emotional, or physiological) and link it to the anger management technique he is most likely to use. Use the **Manage Anger before Problem Solving (MAPS)** handout to include anger cues and anger management techniques in the problem-solving template. Here is an example of a filled-out MAPS form:

How did I know that I was angry?

What was the situation? *My mother told me to get off the phone and my friend overheard it.*

Were there any signs of anger in my body? *For a moment I felt as if the blood was rushing to my face.*

What words ran through my head? *I was gonna say, "Shut up, Mom!"*

What did I do to manage my anger and to cool off?

Breathing, relaxation? *I took a deep breath.*

Calming self-talk? *I thought just calm down, if I yell at her she's not gonna drive me to the mall tonight.*

Distraction? *This whole thing only took a moment so I really did not do anything else.*

5.　***Reinforce the use of appropriate verbal solutions.*** Social skills and communication strategies will be discussed in more depth in Sessions 7–9, but now is a good time to bring up the fact that calmly talking about a problem is usually the best way to find a solution. Children who are prone to physical aggression may have difficulty with verbal skills. They may have difficulty talking about their side of the situation, making verbal requests, using appropriate vocal qualities, or negotiating with others. Consequently, children who don't know what to say may use inappropriate language such as cursing and threatening. Children who tend to be argumentative and talk back to adults may be used to being told that they talk too much. This is also ineffective communication because instead of solving the problem it annoys other people. As part of problem-solving training during this session, it can be helpful to provide the child with a script of what exactly he can say when confronting a particular problem.

Usually the best outcome to a conflict is found when people talk about the problem and solve it together. The relationship may even improve after such a successful interaction. The key word here is talk. Let's say you have a problem with your dad. So you talk about it, solve the problem, and then go fishing together. The outcome is that you solved a problem and you enjoy spending time with each other even more than you did before. Today we spoke about different sides of problem solving, and I can tell you negotiation is the winner. Generally, when you are generating verbal solutions, first think about what you want to say and then think about what effect it will have on the other person. Ask yourself if you should say it. Will it help solve the problem? Will it improve your relationship with this person, or will it hurt your relationship?

5.1. *Practice verbal problem-solving strategies.* Therapists may use the **Words to Express Anger Politely** handout and ask children how they could use some of these polite words in the anger-provoking situations that were reported in this session.

Older children may appreciate an analogy between problem-solving skills discussed in this session and negotiations conducted in the world of politics. Successful negotiations are carried out in a polite and calm voice, and may continue even when several previous attempts at reaching a solution have failed. Role-play an argument the child has frequently with his parents (about chores, computer time, homework). Practice having a conversation about the issues in a way that does not escalate to a confrontation or an argument. Note that swear words, put-downs, and sarcasm are sure barriers to effective communication.

Sarcasm—"You're always right."
Swear words
Put-downs—"You never listen to me."
Dismissive comments—"Whatever."

6. **Summarize the session and assign homework.** The therapist can summarize the session contents by paraphrasing some of the client's relevant comments and by saying:

Today we spoke about the different steps of problem solving. The first step is to know if there is a problem—either for you or for another person. The next step is to think of several solutions to this problem and about the likely consequences of different things that can be done in this problem situation. The final step is to select the best solution and to implement it in a calm tone of voice. We also spoke about how anger can limit our ability to solve problems so that we should first manage anger and then solve the problem.

6.1. **Anger Management Log 5** should be filled out for the next session of the program. The child should record one episode during which he effectively managed his anger and then used a verbal problem-solving strategy.

6.2. *The **PICC** and **MAPS** handouts can be given as an additional homework assignment.* These parallel the **Anger Management Log 5** for this week, but if the child enjoyed these forms during the session, they can be given as part of homework as well.

7.   ***Check in with parent(s).*** At the end of each session, parent(s) or guardian(s) can be invited for a brief check-in to review material of the session, progress during the past week, and the anger management plan for the next week. Ask the parent to give an example of a time when their child was able to engage in appropriate behavior (e.g., walked away from a fight, took out the trash when asked only once) in a situation that could have triggered anger or noncompliance. Ask the child to tell his parents what he learned in session. If needed, therapists may provide two or three bullet points from the session material that resonated most with the child.

Evaluating Consequences

 GOALS

1. Collect homework and review the previous session's material.
2. Introduce consequential thinking.
3. Discuss consequences for other people.
4. Practice consequential thinking.
5. Troubleshoot resistance to problem-solving training.
6. Summarize the session and assign homework.
7. Check in with parent(s).

 HANDOUTS

Problem Identification, Choices, and Consequences (PICC)
Manage Anger before Problem Solving (MAPS)
Fishing Boat
Behavioral Contract

 HOMEWORK

Anger Management Log 6

1.   ***Collect homework and review the previous session's material.***

Last time we spoke about the three steps in problem solving. Do you remember what they are? Did you have a chance to use the **PICC** handout in any of the conflict situations that occurred during the past week?

We also spoke about how anger may interfere with our ability to think about the consequences of our actions. Remember how we practiced the **MAPS** approach to anger management before problem solving? Did you have a chance to use anger management in combination with problem-solving steps?

1.1.   *Review the situation reported in **Anger Management Log 5** and emphasize that there is always more than one way to solve any interpersonal problem. Review solutions generated by the child as part of the problem-solving homework and discuss his rationale for implementing a particular strategy over the others. Hopefully, the child will report being able to successfully negotiate a solution acceptable to all involved parties in a conflict. If not, this could be a good time to model and role-play a verbal strategy.*

2.   ***Introduce consequential thinking.*** The main theme of this session is learning to evaluate multiple consequences of a particular course of action. To begin this section, prompt the child to think back to some of the consequences generated on the **PICC** handout during the last session (or on the homework assignment). If needed, the therapist can review the meaning of the word *consequence*, for example:

Something that happens as a result of what you do. I'd like you to tell me what the word *consequence* means to you—how would you define it?

"Thinking ahead" is another way to refer to this topic, particularly with younger children who may have not learned the word *consequence* yet.

Lead a discussion on the effects of the child's behavior on the outcomes of conflict situations. The simplest way to describe consequences is to divide them into outcomes that are either positive, such as "getting what you want," or negative, such as "getting in trouble." At the same time, a person's behavior may have multiple effects: on his own self-image, on his reputation, on other people's feelings, and on his relationships with others. For example, getting what you want in an argument may also have negative consequences such as feeling guilty and damaging the relationship with the other person involved. Children may not always consider the negative effects of their behavior on others. For example, the child may not immediately see how hurting his parents' feelings in an argument, treating a teacher disrespectfully, or physically hurting a peer in a fight could be viewed as a negative consequence. Therefore, an important aspect of consequential thinking is trying to predict the effect of one's own actions on other people.

When we think about consequences, we think about what the outcomes are for us. Are we going to get in trouble or will we be able to get away with something? We are thinking about the risks and benefits of our actions. But one of the most important consequences of our behavior has to do with its effects on other people. Are they going to like us or hate us as a result of what we've done? It is important to analyze and keep in mind how other people would feel or what they would think about us as an outcome of our actions. You should try to put yourself in the shoes of the other people and think about how your actions will affect them.

The therapist should select some of the previously reported conflict situations and use them to discussion whether or not these situations could have been prevented or resolved by thinking about consequences ahead of time.

2.1. Use the **Fishing Boat** handout to start a discussion about consequences. Give the handout to the child and ask him to decide which items he would keep and which he would throw overboard.

Imagine that you are on a fishing boat that has run into bad weather and engine trouble several miles from shore. The captain has told you that because of the rough weather, the boat needs to be lighter to avoid sinking. You, as a member of the crew, need to decide which items to keep and which items to throw overboard. You are allowed to keep only three items.
Here's a list of the items and their potential uses.

- Box of matches: to help you make a fire for cooking
- Radio (ship to shore):   to try to contact others for help
- Compass: to help you find which direction to go
- Navigational map: to help you find which direction to go
- 10-gallon jug of water: you can't drink water from the ocean/sea
- Signal flares: if help is visible, this can draw attention to you
- Life rafts: if the ship begins to sink, this can keep you from drowning
- 100 feet of rope: by tying yourself to the ship, you can avoid being swept away
- Flashlight: to help you see at night, or to send light signals to shore
- Life jackets: if you fall overboard, this can save you from drowning

Give the child a few minutes to work on the activity, and then discuss his decisions to keep or discard various items in terms of their consequences. Encourage the child to think of multiple consequences for throwing each item overboard. Then talk about how confident he is with his decisions. These are some possible discussion questions:

What was the problem in this situation?

Did thinking about the consequences change your decision about which items to keep? How is this activity relevant to an anger-control program?

This activity can also be used to highlight the difference between the decision making in life-and-death situations versus everyday problems that arise among people. Common problems do not involve the issue of survival, and consequently there is much more room for flexibility in actions and decisions.

3. *Discuss consequences for other people.* One of our study participants shared a relevant observation. His mother was concerned about frequent and what she perceived as "violent" arguments at home. The boy, however, thought that they were just talking. When asked about how he would explain his mother's perception, he said, "I don't think we have too many problems. A problem is when, for instance, someone throws a rock through the window. In our case, it's just like flicking specks of sand against the glass." This was a good starting point to discuss the difference in how the problems were perceived by the boy and his mother. What he thought were specks of sand, his mother saw as rocks through the window.

Ask if the child has noticed if there is anything he says or does that may be annoying to other people, his parents in particular. Therapists should use caution in deciding whether to mention some of the specific complaints they have heard from parents. Try to use open-ended questions and provide praise for thoughtful self-observations.

Have you noticed anything about how you talk or act during conflict?
Do you think there is anything that may be perceived as annoying when you discuss something with your parents (teacher, neighbor, etc.)?
Is there anything you do that may be getting in the way of problem solving?

Then the therapist and the child can choose one of the bad habits the child identifies and develop a behavioral plan and contract for its elimination. A sample **Behavioral Contract** is provided. An example of an "annoying habit" would be: when you are arguing with someone, imitating how he speaks or talking too long to get to the point in a discussion.

4. *Practice consequential thinking.* Recall a typical problem situation that involves a parent or a teacher. Ask the child to generate as many solutions as he can and to identify how the solution might affect the feelings of the other person and his relationship with this person. Also, ask the child to make a prediction about what the other person might do in response to these various solutions. The following questions can be used to guide the discussion:

What would be the consequence of this solution?
How would the person feel if you did this?

What might the person do in response to your behavior?
What else might happen?
What else might the other person do?
What else might the other person feel?

The goal of this activity is to practice consequential thinking in social conflicts and to reinforce the idea that each "solution" has its own consequence. The following conclusion can be drawn from the discussion.

To make a good decision it is necessary to think about all the possible consequences and then choose the solution that would both minimize additional problems and also help you attain your personal goals. Remember that maintaining a positive relationship with another person is also a goal in conflict resolution.

This could be a good place to return to the **Anger Management Logs** and ask the child to reanalyze some of the choices that he made in past conflict situations.

This activity should be repeated for problem solving with peers. If time does not permit additional practice, select the context that is most troublesome for the child. Social problem–solving deficits may vary by context:

- Family: for example, siblings, mother, father, chores.
- School: for example, teachers, schoolmates, in-class, during unsupervised time.
- Community: for example, adults in the mall, police, neighbors.

4.1. *Consequence tic-tac-toe* involves playing tic-tac-toe while thinking about consequences to different problems. Use a board game tic-tac-toe or draw a tic-tac-toe grid on a writing board and discuss the rules as follows:

We will play a game that involves thinking about different consequences for actions in problem situations. I will read a problem [listed below or, alternatively, ask the child to offer a problem] and then we will have to come up with one solution to that problem and at least one consequence. You can go first, and after you come up with a solution and a consequence, you can put an X on the board anywhere you want. Then I will have a turn to think of a solution and a consequence to the problem; if I am able to come up with a *different* solution and consequence, then I will get to choose a place to put an O on the board. Before taking the next turn, everyone has to come up with a new solution.

The following scenarios may be used:

1. A classmate takes your pencil and throws it out the window.
2. A classmate starts teasing you and calling you names.
3. You find out that a classmate was spreading a bad rumor about you.

Play a few rounds, providing social reinforcement for appropriate solutions. Lead the child to a better understanding of the benefits associated with prosocial behavior.

5. ***Troubleshoot resistance to problem-solving training.*** One of the challenges of talking about the negative consequences is that the child may insist that he does not care what the consequences are, which may be the case with some long-standing conflicts. In our work we found it easier to switch gears and move on to a different topic rather than trying to convince a child that he does care about consequences. A broader discussion about consequences in general may have a better chance of finding a receptive audience if it does not run directly up against a particularly challenging problem. Whatever the problem, the therapist may revisit it at a later point with a different anger management technique.

Underestimating the likelihood of negative consequences of particular high-risk behaviors is another issue therapists may encounter with some children. Particularly in adolescents, if there is a risk of problem behaviors such as drinking and driving, having unprotected sex, participating in gang fights, and the like, this has to be addressed in supervision and may become a separate focus of clinical attention that goes beyond the scope of this manual.

6. ***Summarize the session and assign homework.*** Summarize the parts of the session that were most relevant to the child. For example:

Today we spoke about consequences. There is more to it than just staying out of trouble. Our actions can affect our reputation, friendships, other people's feelings, and what other people think about us. So it is important to consider all the different effects that our actions may have.

6.1. **Anger Management Log 6** should be filled out for the next session of the program. The child should be asked to record one episode from the following week in which he is able to effectively manage a problem situation by thinking about the consequences of his actions in problem situations ("think-ahead" method).

7. ***Check in with parent(s).*** At the end of each session, parent(s) or guardian(s) can be invited for a brief check-in to review material of the session, progress during the past week, and the anger management plan for the next week. Ask the parent to give an example of a time when their child was able to engage in appropriate behavior (e.g., walked away from a fight, took out the trash when asked only once) in a situation that could have triggered anger or noncompliance. Ask the child to tell parents what he learned in session. If needed, therapists may provide two or three bullet points from the session material that resonated most with the child.

MODULE 3

SOCIAL SKILLS

Developing a Coping Template for Peer Provocation

 GOALS

1. Collect homework and review the previous session's material.
2. Introduce social skills training.
3. Define and discuss assertive behavior and de-escalation.
4. Develop a coping template for peer provocation.
5. Practice assertiveness skills.
6. Discuss nonverbal aspects of social interaction.
7. Summarize the session and assign homework.
8. Check in with parent(s).

 MATERIALS

Dominos, playing cards, or Jenga; a mirror

HANDOUTS

Role-Play Practice
Three Ways of Acting

 HOMEWORK

Anger Management Log 7a (Assertive Response to Teasing)
Anger Management Log 7b (Ignoring Teasing)

1.   ***Collect homework and review the previous session's material.*** Review **Anger Management Log 6** from last week and provide praise for reported successful problem solving. Ask the child what he remembers about the material covered in the last session.

> **Note to Therapists:** Problem-solving and cognitive restructuring techniques may not resonate with each child. If the child does not remember much about the problem-solving module of the training, it could be a sign that other anger management skills could be more relevant. If the treatment is done as part of a research study, the therapist may review the content of the previous session to fulfill the requirements of treatment fidelity. If the treatment is provided as a clinical service, the therapist may skip the review and move on to the new material.

The problem-solving portion of the program can be summarized in the following way:

Successful problem-solving strategies allow us to do the right thing, to resolve problems, and to stay out of trouble. Avoiding fighting and name calling is also part of successful problem solving. In other words, we can judge behavior by its outcomes. Last time we spoke about how our actions in conflict situations can affect our reputation, our friendships, and other people's feelings. Our actions can also get us into trouble. It is important to consider the different consequences that our behaviors may have.

The second important point we discussed is that our beliefs may influence our judgment and behavior in conflict situations. It is helpful to be able to examine our own beliefs (self-disputation), before we act on them.

2.   ***Introduce social skills training.*** The purpose of the remaining sessions is to select and practice anger management and problem-solving strategies that have worked well for a particular child. The goal of this session is to come up with a predetermined course of action that can defuse a peer provocation. Therapists can employ the feedback from the child on the usefulness of material covered so far and use it to build a template of coping skills for the most common problem situations that this child has encountered over the course of the program. The following script can be used to introduce this concept to the child:

Everyone has conflicts sometimes, with their friends, their brothers or sisters, teachers, or parents. Sometimes what we do in such situations may make things worse. We don't say the right thing; we raise our voice; we have an angry look on our face. Even though we might know what the right thing to do is, we still don't act in our best interests. Sometimes it seems as if words come out of our mouths when we don't even mean to say them. Then we are surprised when we find ourselves in heated arguments or fights.

Particularly when we are angry, we may yell and scream, or even push and hit. When we do things like that, we can get ourselves into trouble.

The purpose of the next three sessions of this program is to practice some of the skills that we covered so far with the goal that using these skills becomes almost automatic. Then if you are in a situation that makes you angry or upset, these skills can help you manage the conflict before it gets out of control. Some of the most common, frustrating events that you mentioned before were [include this child's common anger-provoking events]. Let's practice handling some of these problems.

2.1. *Modeling and role play are the key techniques for Sessions 7–9.* Short role plays were also used in the previous session, but longer role plays are useful to rehearse social skills techniques. The child can be reminded about the use of role plays as follows:

Role playing is similar to acting, like in the movies or the theater. We will role-play various conflict situations so that we can practice skills that can help to resolve problems.

A simple role play can be modeled by using a prototypical student–teacher situation (see the **Role-Play Practice** handout). Therapist should assume the student's role and reenact three types of responses to a teacher's reprimand. The child should be the teacher in the following situation:

You are Mr. Smith, a teacher in a junior high school. Your student, me, does not pay attention in class.

CHILD (*acting as teacher*): How many times have I told you to pay attention?

Scenario 1 (disrespectful response)

THERAPIST (*acting as student*): I am listening; you are always picking on me!

Scenario 2 (passive response)

THERAPIST: (*Mumbles incoherently and looks down.*)

Scenario 3 (appropriate response)

THERAPIST: Sorry, Mr. Smith. It won't happen again.

Discuss the role play in terms of the likelihood that the child would use the three different ways of responding in real life. Then ask the child to role-play how he would respond to the teacher's reprimand.

3. ***Define and discuss assertive behavior and de-escalation.*** Assertive behavior refers to confident and direct communication, claiming one's rights in a way that reduces the intensity of a conflict. Assertive behavior is an appropriate response to provocation, but it is also aimed at reducing the chances of escalation of the problem. To contrast assertive behavior with aggressive behavior, it could be helpful to draw a diagram of a common sequence of events—*Provocation → Aggressive Behavior → Confrontation*—and use it as a visual aid. The therapist can use one of the situations reported by the child to illustrate this sequence.

Often our anger response is out of proportion to its provocation. For example, if someone looks at you the wrong way, you curse them out. If someone curses at you, you punch them in the face. That's how problems start: everyone reacts just a little stronger than his provocateur, and in a few seconds, there is a fight. The key word of today's lesson is de-escalation. Imagine that your reactions in conflict are like walking down stairs: every step brings down the level of anger in the situation. You can diffuse and resolve the problem before it goes through the roof.

Define the terms "passive," "aggressive," and "assertive" behavioral responses to provocation. Write these on the board and discuss them briefly; the **Three Ways of Acting** handout can also be used for illustration.

> **Passive**: doing nothing when something bad happens to you.
> **Aggressive**: fighting or yelling back when something happens.
> **Assertive**: talking the problem out and finding a solution.

If the word "assertive" is new to younger children, help them see the distinction between assertiveness and aggression by emphasizing that assertive behavior allows people to solve problems without resorting to fighting and arguing; rather, it helps people find a way to talk things out. If the child has a tendency to talk back too much, the distinction should be made between "talking" and "arguing." Ask the child to think of an example of when he has acted in an assertive manner.

3.1. The following story can be used to *illustrate the difference between passive, aggressive, and assertive behavior.*

Anthony is in the fifth grade and usually no one bothers him at school. Anthony likes his science classes and he also enjoys playing with other kids during recess. However, there is another kid in Anthony's class who started to pick on Anthony and call him "little baby." Every time this boy, whose name was Mitchell, would run into Anthony after class or during recess, he would say, "Hey, little baby, you are such a little baby." One day Anthony got tired of this. He pushed Mitchell down and kicked him in the face. Mitchell started to cry and a teacher who was passing down the hallway took Anthony to the principal's office.

Ask the child if Anthony's behavior was passive, aggressive, or assertive and ask what else Anthony could have done instead. Group responses into aggressive (e.g.,

"He could have just pushed him away," "He did not have to kick him," or "He could have waited for him in a place where no one would see them and then beat him up") and assertive (e.g., "He could have told him to stop bothering him" or "He could have tried to become friends with him"). Role-play assertive behavior where the therapist is Mitchell and the child is Anthony.

4.   ***Develop a coping template for peer provocation.*** Ask the child to recall several peer conflicts and, if possible, group these situations into categories. Some of the likely categories are being teased or "disrespected" and having one's property damaged.

Let's review some of the problems that you might run into with the other kids at school. What do they do that ticks you off? Let's get a few typical situations written down and then we can role-play what can be done in each of these situations.

For example, one girl who participated in this treatment, let's call her Sasha, reported the following situation. Sasha was in class trying to pay attention to the lesson while two other girls were talking with each other in the back of the room. After missing several of the teacher's points because of their whispering, Sasha turned around and said, "Quiet." One of the other girls responded, "Don't make me slap you." Sasha banged her fist on the desk and gave the girls a long, angry stare. At this point the teacher noticed the commotion and scolded Sasha for causing a disruption.

In our discussion of this situation, Sasha came up with three strategies for dealing with this problem if it were to happen again. First, we role-played saying "not cool" in response to a threatening comment—this is the example of a coping template for peer provocation. Second, we agreed that a better strategy for handling a situation when someone is talking during the class is to tell the teacher. Finally, a preventive strategy was suggested: Sasha can ask the teacher for permission to sit closer to the front of the class and farther away from the kids who can be distracting.

4.1.   *Address teasing and name calling.* Ask the child to make a list of what other children might say that would make him angry and ask which verbal provocations can be ignored and which cannot be ignored.

> **Can be ignored**: not worth paying attention to (e.g., when someone is joking).
> **Can be responded to assertively**: the person is saying something inappropriate and should
>   be asked to stop.

The therapist should help the child identify which provocations can be ignored and ask the child which techniques (relaxation, self-talk, etc.) he could use to make it easier to ignore these provocations during the next week. For provocations that cannot be ignored assertive responses are described below. If the child reports clear acts of ridicule or intimidation, he and his parents may be invited to discuss whether these peer provocations represent incidents of bullying that need to be addressed by the school administration. A detailed discussion of bullying prevention is outside the scope of this book, but excellent resources for therapists and families are available (Swearer, Espelage, & Napolitano, 2009).

4.2.   [Optional Activity] *The barb exposure technique can be used to desensitize the child to common verbal provocations.* This technique involves presenting an unpleasant statement to a child while the child uses a particular anger management strategy. This technique has been used with adult men (Grodnitzky & Tafrate, 2000; Tafrate & Kassinove, 1998), but in our experience it can be used with children, with caution, in certain instances. Therapists should use this technique only if they are confident that the levels of induced anger can be successfully diffused before the end of the session. Good clinical judgment and experience are needed to select and deliver the barbs in a way that elicits anger, on the one hand, while at the same time ensuring that the child can diffuse the anger and not leave the session feeling offended, on the other hand. A good treatment alliance is another prerequisite for using the barb exposure technique. The therapist may explain the rationale to the child in the following way:

There is one method that can help you become less affected when people tease you or call you names. Let's write down a few mean things that people have said to you in the past. Then we can role-play the situation; I will say these mean things out loud, and you will ignore them. The rationale behind this technique is that by exposing yourself to the names people call you or mean things they say here, where it's safe, you will be less sensitive to the real provocations. You can think of it like a flu shot, which makes you immune to the flu. Our goal is to try to make you immune to the mean things people say.

The *in vivo* version of this procedure can be implemented in two ways. First, the child can be asked to use reminders, such as "Ignore this" or "I don't care," when the therapist delivers the barbs. A second approach is to ask the child to engage in an attention-absorbing activity, such as building a house from a deck of cards or building a tower with dominos or Jenga blocks. The benefit of the second approach is that it can be used to demonstrate that by concentrating one's attention on something besides the barbs, it becomes possible to ignore these annoying provocations.

5.   ***Practice assertiveness skills.*** Negotiating or talking out a problem can be the best problem-solving strategy. De-escalating assertion, or increasing the number and the emphasis of requests for someone to stop a provocative behavior, can be employed if one simple request does not work.

Unfortunately, sometimes ignoring another person does not stop this person from saying nasty things over and over again. In such cases we need to firmly tell that person to stop. However, we also need to make sure we don't get into more trouble or into another fight. For example, can you think of something to say if someone in your class, another guy your age, starts picking on you and calling you names?

Try to get several alternative solutions in response to this question and then model and role-play assertive responses such as these:

You can say "Stop bothering me, I don't like when you call me this." If the person continues, you can say, "If you don't stop, I won't talk to you anymore." If this person continues to bother you or if he tries to pick a fight, you can say "I am not going to get in trouble because of you. If you don't stop, I will tell the teacher."

Help the child identify one assertive response that he thinks will work best for him and write it down on an index card; this will be the reminder for the coping response the child can use if he is teased by his peers during the next week.

5.1. *Discuss the importance of using "I" statements when making a direct request for change.* This communication tactic reduces the accusatory tone of requests.

Making requests is not always hard to do. Keep in mind, though, that it is important to make requests in a nice manner. For example, instead of cursing back at this other guy, you should say, "It bothers me when you do that. Please, stop it."

Let's consider a hypothetical situation. Your older friend, who is also taller than you, calls you "Shorty," and you'd rather be called by your real name.

FRIEND: Hey, Shorty, did you get out of class early?

YOU: Listen, can you call me by my real name?

FRIEND: What's wrong with Shorty?

YOU: I just like to be called by my name.

FRIEND: Well, I didn't know it bothered you. I call a lot of people Shorty.

YOU: I know I'm short, but it's not the most important thing about me, and I wish you would call me by my real name.

FRIEND: That's cool.

YOU: Thanks.

5.2. *Role-play real-life scenarios.* The therapist can use scenarios from the **Anger Management Logs** to role-play verbal responses to provocations that the child has encountered in real life. It is helpful to first write down the description of the situation and a script of the assertive communication that can be reenacted in the role play. The child can be asked to play the provocateur and then himself. Some of the most common verbal provocations include negative comments about clothes, looks, and abilities (athletics, academics, etc.). We recommend avoiding profanities with sexual connotations and racial or religious slurs in this activity. However, it is important to solicit from the child examples of language that is considered insulting in his peer environment.

6.   ***Discuss nonverbal aspects of social interaction.*** It is not only what we say that can provoke others, but also how we say it. Therapists can use their acting abilities to dramatize the differences between neutral or positive nonverbal behavior and threatening or provocative nonverbal behavior using posture, gestures, facial expressions, and tones of voice. For example, finger pointing, head shaking, and scowling are common nonverbal signs that accompany verbal confrontation. Eye rolling and sighing can signal disapproval and be perceived as provocative.

Have the child practice saying a neutral phrase such as "Have a nice day" in a loud voice and with an intense stare, eyebrows pulled together. Then have the child practice making assertive statements such as "Don't call me that" and "I asked you to stop it" in a calm tone of voice and with a neutral facial expression. Discuss and role-play other elements of nonverbal behavior. For example, personal space can be discussed in the following manner:

It is important that we keep our distance from another person when talking. Make sure you always stay at least one arm's length away when you talk to someone. This is another way to be assertive without being aggressive and getting into another person's face.

The following are helpful key points about assertive nonverbal behavior:

Use a *calm voice* (i.e., don't yell).
Use an arm's length of *personal space* (i.e., don't get into another person's face).
Don't make threatening *gestures* (i.e., pointing fingers).
Maintain *eye contact.*

6.1.   *We often infer the emotions of other people by observing their facial expressions, and then we might reciprocate their affect.* When someone smiles at us, we smile in return. By the same token, when someone frowns, we are likely to think he is angry or his intentions are hostile, and we react accordingly. One of the reasons that children are labeled as "angry" is because they look angry. Therefore, teaching the child to pay attention to his facial expressions and learn to modulate facial expressions of anger can be a helpful social skill. Practice assertive responses to verbal provocations while maintaining a neutral facial expression. If there isn't already a mirror in the office, consider bringing in a hand-held one so the child can see his own expressions.

7.   ***Summarize the session and assign homework.*** Ask the child to recall the main points and discuss how the session material may be relevant to his current anger triggers. Review productive comments that the child might have made during the session. A brief summary can be offered:

Today we spoke about acting in a way that can solve problems and not lead to any trouble. We call this assertive communication, and it helps us to talk in a firm but not threatening way. If a peer bothers or provokes you, the first thing you need to do is to decide if you can ignore it. If this is a situation in which you feel you need to stick up for yourself, you should act in an assertive manner by using words to convince this person to stop bothering you, maintaining a calm voice and a calm expression. If the person refuses to leave you alone, you can calmly tell him that you're going to let a teacher (or another adult) know what's happening.

7.1. *Assign **Anger Management Logs** (7a and 7b) for next week.* Explain that the goal is to practice two skills: ignoring provocations and using assertive communication. Ideally, this session should result in the development and rehearsal of a behavioral response to some ongoing problem situation with peers. Encourage the child to use the **Anger Management Logs** to record the results of practicing these behavioral responses in the context of ongoing conflict situations.

8. ***Check in with parent(s).*** At the end of each session, parent(s) or guardian(s) can be invited for a brief check-in to review material of the session, progress during the past week, and the anger management plan for the next week. Ask the parent to give an example of a time when their child was able to engage in appropriate behavior (e.g., walked away from a fight, took out the trash when asked only once) in a situation that could have triggered anger or noncompliance. Ask the child to tell his parents what he learned in session. If needed, therapists may provide two or three bullet points from the session material that resonated most with the child.

Assertiveness Training

 GOALS

1. Collect homework and review the previous session's material.
2. Discuss fairness and rights.
3. Role-play social skills when rights have been violated.
4. Practice active listening skills.
5. Develop a coping template for dealing with accusation.
6. Summarize the session and assign homework.
7. Check in with parent(s).

 HANDOUTS

The Bill of Rights
Three Steps of Active Listening

☑ **HOMEWORK**

Anger Management Log 8a (Assertiveness Skills)
Anger Management Log 8b (Dealing with Accusation)
Daily Anger Monitoring Log (optional, same as in Session 1)

1. **Collect homework and review the previous session's material.**

Last time we talked about situations when other people call us names, tease, or bother us in different ways. We learned that it is important to be able to ignore these people and to ask them to stop, politely, without getting ourselves in trouble.

1.1. *Review the situations described in **Anger Management Logs 7a and 7b.*** Inquire about the child's experience with techniques covered in the last session: ignoring trivial provocations, making verbal requests, using "I" statements, and paying attention to nonverbal behavior.

1.2. *If the child did not use assertive coping strategies in the situations described in the homework assignments, briefly discuss and model assertive responses.* After assertive problem-solving strategies have been demonstrated, role-play specific verbal and nonverbal elements of the situation.

2. **Discuss fairness and rights.**

> **Note to Therapists:** Assertiveness training is based on the assumption that people should stand up for their rights and not tolerate the injustices of the world. In psychotherapy, assertiveness training has been used for all kinds of purposes. For example, people who are too humble may be actually taught to get in touch with their anger and rectify the wrongs that were done to them. Individuals who are too angry may be taught to express their anger without encroaching on the right of others not to be insulted. The assertiveness training movement has left a legacy of two basic assumptions that are very relevant to CBT for anger and aggression:
>
> 1. A person should express his or her feelings without hurting another person's feelings.
> 2. People should stand up for their rights without intruding on the rights of others.

Being able to stick up for yourself with authority figures requires a great deal of social skill. Competent execution of these skills implies that we are aware of our rights and have a sense of fairness. Rights include various freedoms and entitlements. Fairness means that people are treated equally and receive what they deserve. The issue of rights and fairness is also linked to anger experience because people tend to get angry when their rights are violated or when they are treated unfairly.

Unfair treatment is a common occurrence in a child's life. In the problem-solving module of the treatment, the focus was on teaching the child to sort out events that were in fact unfair from those that may have only been perceived as unfair because of cognitive biases. The goal of this section is to create a coping template for appropriate, assertive actions when the child's rights are objectively violated. If this is the case, his anger would be a correct emotional response to the situation and the child should act on this anger ("Don't let it slide") in order to rectify the injustice. These actions should be legal, socially appropriate, and considerate of the transgressor's feelings.

Underscore the connection of social skills training with the problem-solving skills by pointing out that anger often involves misattributions of fairness and blame. Therefore, using socially skilled behavior to rectify objective injustices should be preceded by a careful problem-solving analysis of the situation.

Everyone has the right to be treated fairly and with respect. People often get angry when they feel that they are being treated unfairly. For example, if your sister gets to watch television and you have to do your homework, it might feel unfair. Or, if you are punished for something you did not do, it is unfair. Of course, we have already spoken about considering other people's goals and intentions in order to understand whether something is fair or not. We learned to use problem-solving skills to evaluate what's actually going on—not just from our point of view, but from the point of view of others as well. But when something is really unfair, that's when you should act to right the wrong. Can you think of a situation in which you were treated unfairly?

Being angry is OK when your rights are violated. You also want to make sure that when your rights are being violated you can stand up for yourself. However, you have to be able to do it without hurting others.

Ask the child to fill out **The Bill of Rights** handout. For example, Feindler and Ecton (1986) suggested a list of five rights that can be helpful in discussing assertive communication with aggressive youth: the right to be listened to, the right to explain one's side of the story, the right to own property, the right not to be insulted, and the right not to be hurt.

Ask the child if he can tell how and by whom each of these five rights was violated in this vignette:

John was brought to the principal's office for throwing food at Howie during lunch. Without even listening to any explanations, the principal sent John to detention. However, Howie had been the one to start it by throwing a milk carton at John.

Correct responses:

The right to be listened to: John's right was violated when the principal refused to listen.

The right to explain one's side of the story: Again, John's right was violated when the principal refused to let John present his side of what happened.

The right to own property: Not applicable to this situation.

The right not to be insulted: John's right was violated when Howie threw a milk carton at him. But Howie's right was also violated because John threw food back at Howie.

The right not to be hurt: Even though this situation might have started as a play food fight, it is conceivable that it might have gotten out of control and progressed to a real fight in which John and Howie could have been hurt.

3. ***Role-play social skills when rights have been violated.***

Unfortunately, the teasing we discussed last time is not the only bad thing that can happen to us. Sometimes friends borrow your things and then break them or don't return them. Sometimes teachers give you an unfairly low grade. Sometimes parents don't let you watch your favorite TV show when they previously told you that you could. Can you recall similar situations or other examples of unfair things that have happened to you?

Have the child recall specific examples of being treated unfairly and use social skills to role-play advocating for oneself. Using one of the above examples, or an example the child comes up with, elicit the three types of responses from the child. Discuss the differences between the three ways of handling the situation and then role-play the assertive scenario.

Passive: letting someone take away your rights and doing nothing in response.
Aggressive: demanding your rights with no regard for the other person's rights.
Assertive: standing up for your rights but respecting other people's rights as well.

Practice using a firm and unemotional tone of voice and short, direct statements to formulate a request. Highlight that this strategy can be used in provoking situations that cannot be simply ignored.

Let's pretend that someone has taken your book. One thing you can do is keep repeating, "Please give me my book back," until your book is returned. Make sure you repeat your demand in the same calm and monotone voice until you get what you need.

This technique should first be modeled by the therapist. Then the therapist should take something that belongs to the child (such as an iPod), and ask the child to practice asking for this thing back. Modeling and feedback can be provided to illustrate various helpful and not helpful verbal and nonverbal elements that can be part of this communication.

4. ***Practice active listening skills.***

Note to Therapists: One of the less obvious but critical elements in the sequence of social interaction is listening. Social skills that might be trained as part of various treatments can be grouped in two broad categories: macroskills and microskills. Macroskills are the general behavioral strategies for particular social situations, such as asking a favor or asking a fried to go to the movies. Microskills are the building blocks in a chain of a complex social response. Examples of microskills are facial expressions (e.g., smiling), motor behaviors (e.g., slouching), and vocal qualities (e.g., mumbling). These microskills, which can be employed in active listening, constitute the nuances of social behavior. When observed by another person, these can be powerful messages about motivation and emotion. When accompanied by eye contact—the facial expression that signals attention—listening can be a powerful social skill for preventing conflicts.

Present the topic of active listening to the child:

Conflicts and problems often arise because people don't listen to each other. Sometimes we can't even hear what another person has just said because we were thinking about our own comeback line. If you take time to listen, chances are the conflict can be prevented altogether. If we are angry at a person, listening to him becomes difficult because anger depletes our attention.

Ask if this makes sense to the child and, if needed, clarify with this example.

For example, if a teacher accuses you of something that you did not do, your first natural response would be to say something in defense of yourself, such as "I didn't do it." However, responses like that just make the situation worse because they are perceived as a disagreement. In fact, you are disagreeing with your teacher. Imagine that you say something like "What do you mean?" This will probably give you time to figure out what's going on. The teacher will have a chance to explain what happened, and as he or she does so, the problem may become clarified.

Ask the child to think of some reasons why listening to another person during a conflict situation can be beneficial.

There are three steps in the active listening sequence, which can be discussed using the **Three Steps of Active Listening** handout as a visual aid. The three steps are:

Listen carefully to what is being said.
Repeat the statement back to the person.
Clarify what is the problem in the situation.

4.1. *The first step in active listening is simply to pay attention to the other person when he is talking. The second step is to clarify the point that the other person is making.* This can be done either by asking a question or paraphrasing what you've heard him say. Therapists should be aware that some children may have a tendency to repeat others in order to annoy them. In addition, if a child were to use this approach in the wrong circumstances, it might be perceived as "acting smart" or "having an attitude." There are also less common circumstances that should also be taken into account; for example, a child with Tourette syndrome may have a symptom called echolalia, in which he compulsively repeats what he has heard. In these cases, the active listening training can be modified or skipped altogether. However, for the majority of children this is a helpful skill to have in the repertoire of social skills for dealing with disruptive behavior.

There are times when we may not pay full attention to a conversation we're having. If someone asks us to repeat what he just said when we haven't been listening, we would have no idea what to say. It can be helpful to clarify the main point being made by another person. Particularly in communication with parents and teachers, a calm, sincere, and interested facial expression can communicate that you care, appreciate, and acknowledge what they're saying. Avoid smiling or looking angry when a teacher or a parent is expressing anger. If you do, you may upset them even more by making then feel that you are not taking the issue seriously.

Practice active listening with the child using the list below. You can read each phrase and ask the child to repeat it.

Statement samples	Sample responses
1. I got an A on the last math test.	1. You got an A on your last math test.
2. Can I borrow your eraser for a minute?	2. You want to borrow my eraser?
3. Give me my pencil back or I will tell the teacher.	3. You want me to give you this pencil?
4. Three boys were playing catch in the backyard.	4. Some boys were playing in the backyard.

4.2. *The final step of active listening—clarification of the point—means telling the person how you understand the gist of the problem.*

After the other person has told you about the problem, even if you are able to repeat his statement back to him, you may still need more information. If you're able to clarify what's going on, you can be sure that both people are talking about the same thing. Once the problem is clear, you can use all the problem-solving skills that we have been learning in this program.

Here is an example of a hypothetical active listening exchange role-played between the therapist and the child:

THERAPIST: You know, I wish you would pay more attention to what I am saying here.

CHILD: Would you like me to pay more attention to what you are saying?

THERAPIST: Yes. And would you also stop playing with your video game while we're talking.

CHILD: Are you saying that I should turn off my game and listen to what you're saying?

THERAPIST: Now you've got it.

5. ***Develop a coping template for dealing with accusation.*** One of the most frequent causes of anger is being accused, blamed, or criticized, especially when one is accused of something for the wrong reasons. Even when the blame is well deserved, an argument may follow. The therapist should distinguish between these two types of situations: being accused for a good reason and being accused because of misunderstanding.

Often people accuse us of different things that we did not do. This could be a mistake, a misunderstanding, or some other unfortunate circumstance. For example, you might be accused of cheating on a test, while in reality you did not cheat. Or, you may be accused of starting a fight while you really had just been defending yourself. Your parents may accuse you of messing up a room while it might have been your brother or sister who did it. In any event, we have to be able to explain ourselves without exploding in anger when we're accused of something.

Ask the child to provide an example of being accused of something by mistake.

When someone accuses you of something that you didn't do, you need to be able to explain it calmly rather than angrily. Keep in mind that something bad has happened to whoever is accusing you and this person may be upset. Remember our discussion about acting without thinking? Take a minute to recall the Stop & Think technique. This person might be acting inappropriately toward you, but you can give him some help to figure things out. For example, let's imagine you picked up your friend's pen from under the desk to give it back to him, but instead of thanking you, your friend yells, "You broke my favorite pen!"

Discuss how to handle this situation using active listening skills: (1) Listen carefully, (2) repeat what you heard, and (3) clarify the situation. For example:

FRIEND: You broke my favorite pen! [accusation]

YOU: Your pen is broken? [clarification of the problem]

FRIEND: Yeah, it's broken, look at this! [stating the problem without casting blame]

YOU: Maybe it can be fixed? [not getting confrontational]

FRIEND: No, it can't. I really loved this pen. [taking a few seconds to calm down]

YOU: Look, I just picked it up from the floor. I did not break it. [providing explanation]

FRIEND: It's OK. I can get myself another one. [getting control of his emotions]

YOU: Well, sorry about your pen. [acting nice]

5.1. *Role-play active listening skills in a situation of being wrongfully accused,* either from the list below or from reports of real-life situations. Provide corrective feedback and reinforcement for using the three steps of active listening.

You are playing checkers with a friend, and he accuses you of cheating.
Your teacher accuses you of talking in class.
Someone took your friend's textbook and he thinks it was you.

5.2. *Practice making a sincere apology.* Of course, if we are caught with "our hand in the cookie jar," the best way to reduce the victim's anger is to repair the damage and to apologize. Being able to apologize politely is also a social skill that may be relevant to children who participate in this treatment. Like paying a compliment, apologizing politely does not come naturally to everyone. The therapist may briefly discuss why it is a good idea to apologize when you did something wrong. Ask the child to think of reasons why it is a good idea to apologize and write these reasons on the board—for example: "Apologizing ends the problem," "It is the right thing to do," "It makes you a nice person."

Role-play apologizing using either real-life or hypothetical scenarios. Model appropriate nonverbal behaviors such as eye contact and tone of voice. To begin, the therapist can dramatize the following script.

CHILD: Hey, give me my book back, I need it!

THERAPIST: You need your book? [demonstrating appropriate eye contact and body language]

CHILD: You took my book. Can I have it back? [raising voice]

THERAPIST: Oh, I didn't realize it was yours. [still holding on to the book]

CHILD: It's OK. We can use it together.

THERAPIST: I'm sorry. Here you go.

Practice offering an apology for some of the common situations that the child encounters at home or in school. Provide feedback and reinforce assertive verbal and nonverbal responses.

6. **Summarize the session and assign homework.** Ask the child to recall the main points of the session and discuss how this material may be relevant to his current anger situations. A brief summary can be offered:

Today we spoke about the difference between situations that can be ignored and situations that require actions. We described these situations as unjust or unfair. We also spoke about assertive behavior. We covered active listening and also practiced being assertive in making a request without showing anger. Finally, we spoke about different things to do when someone blames you for something. Here the important skill is to listen to the person without escalating the situation. If there was a misunderstanding and you did not do anything wrong, calmly clarify the situation. If you actually did do something wrong, offer to fix the problem and then apologize.

6.1.   Ask the child to hold onto the **Three Steps of Active Listening** handout and use these steps at home and at school.

6.2.   **Anger Management Logs 8a (Assertiveness Skills)** and **8b (Dealing with Accusation)** should be filled out for the next session for the situations in which the child was able to successfully use any of the skills covered in this session.

6.3.   At the end of Session 8, the optional **Daily Anger Monitoring Log** can be introduced or reintroduced if the child has used this optional assignment at the beginning of the treatment. The daily log asks the child to record and briefly describe all incidents of anger that occur before the next session. This assignment can be also repeated after the ninth session in order to provide additional material for the review during the last, 10th session. It can be also informative to compare the logs from the first 2 weeks of treatment with the logs from the last 2 weeks of treatment.

7.   ***Check in with parent(s).*** At the end of each session, parent(s) or guardian(s) can be invited for a brief check-in to review material of the session, progress during the past week, and the anger management plan for the next week. Ask the parent to give an example of a time when their child was able to engage in appropriate behavior in a situation that could have triggered anger or noncompliance. Ask the child to tell his parents what he learned in session. If needed, therapists may provide two or three bullet points from the session material that resonated most with the child.

Social Skills for Conflict Resolution with Adults

 GOALS

1. Collect homework and review the previous session's material.
2. Develop a coping template for conflicts with adults.
3. Discuss situations that lead to conflicts at home.
4. Practice monitoring poor communication habits.
5. Practice explaining one's role in a conflict situation.
6. Summarize the session and assign homework.
7. Check in with parent(s).

 MATERIALS

Index cards

HANDOUTS

Home Situations Questionnaire
Home Situation Problem Solving
Behavioral Contract
Communication Habits

HOMEWORK

Home Situation Problem Solving
Anger Management Log 9
Daily Anger Monitoring Log (optional, same as in Session 1)

1. ***Collect homework and review the previous session's material.*** Because this session deals with parent–child conflicts, therapists can ask the parents to fill out the **Home Situations Questionnaire** (HSQ) at the beginning of the session. This questionnaire can be used to identify situations that lead to conflicts at home. As the parents work on the HSQ, the therapist may proceed with the review of the last session's material with the child. Several minutes can be taken at the beginning of the session to meet with both patent and child in order to identify several conflict situations that can be discussed in the session. After that the parent can be asked to wait outside and rejoin for a check-in at the end of the session.

    Last time we talked about assertive behavior in situations where our rights have been violated. For example, if you are angry about something, being assertive means expressing your anger in a socially appropriate way. Did anything happen last week that required you to be assertive and stand up for your rights?

    Then we spoke about active listening. This is a technique that involves listening to another person, restating what you heard, and then summarizing your understanding of the problem. Were you able to apply any of these skills in the conflict situations of the past week?

    We also spoke about dealing with situations in which someone blames or accuses you for some reason. The way to deal with such situations is first to clarify who caused the problem and then act accordingly. For example, you can either clarify that the problem was not your fault or, if it was, apologize and offer a solution. Were there any situations during this past week that required you to use this skill of dealing with accusation?

1.1. *Review Anger Management Logs 8a and 8b.* If the child did not use assertive coping strategies, provide corrective feedback and model a more appropriate behavior.

1.2. *Review the optional Daily Anger Monitoring Log, if completed.* Ask if the child remembered to include all significant anger episodes for the week. Several minutes can be taken to add the episodes that were missed at home. This form can be used to give the child feedback during the last session of this program.

2. ***Develop a coping template for conflicts with adults.*** First, discuss the reported conflicts involving authority figures (parents, teachers, etc.).

    As we are growing up, we all have to deal with people who are in positions of authority, who are responsible for us, such as parents, teachers, coaches, bosses, and so forth. Sometimes it is difficult to deal with those who have authority over us. These people often demand our respect, which often means we need to treat them differently than we treat our friends. Learning how to deal with those in authority is important if you want to avoid arguments and stay out of trouble. For example, if a teacher asks you, "Why aren't you in your class? Recess is over," and you snap back, "I'll get to class when

I want to," you will get into even more trouble than if you had simply answered "I know I'm late, I'm on my way to class." It is important to realize that what we say, how we say it, and to whom we say it can sometimes get us in trouble.

The anger management and problem-solving skills discussed so far are also applicable to conflicts with adults. If parent–child conflict is the main area of concern, this session can be conducted with parent and child together. Child noncompliance and disruptive behavior are also addressed in treatments known as "parent management training," where the parents rather than the children receive the intervention. In this CBT manual, the time spent with the parents and direct teaching of skills to the parents is limited because this is a child-focused treatment, and excellent parent management training resources are available elsewhere (see Introduction for details).

The therapist should be careful when addressing parent–child conflicts that are chronic or that stem from possible comorbid conditions such as ADHD and obsessive–compulsive disorder. For example, one child who was in this program also had compulsive washing rituals that lasted for nearly 2 hours every day. Consequently, being late to school and leaving a mess in the bathroom always resulted in arguments at home. Clearly, treatment of compulsive symptoms is well beyond the scope of this manual. However, learning to talk about the problem situations caused by these symptoms without excessive anger was helpful in reducing the number and intensity of conflicts.

2.1. *Give an example of a response to a conflict with a parent.*

Imagine you went to spend an afternoon with some friends and agreed to be home by 4:00 P.M. since your family had early dinner plans. Then you lost track of time and did not get home until 4:45 P.M.

Let's role-play how you and your parents could have discussed this situation. I will be you and you will be your parent (mother or father, whomever you prefer).

After conducting a brief role play, offer an example of an apology that could have diffused this situation.

PARENT: You were supposed to be home by 4:00—you are 45 minutes late! You are going to lose your weekend privileges for 2 weeks.

YOU: I'm sorry I was late. I know you were counting on my being home at 4:00. I'm sorry you had to wait for me for dinner. I should have paid more attention to what time it was, but I didn't.

PARENT: That's right; you let me down! You are going to have to learn how to be more responsible.

YOU: I know. I will try to remember better next time.

After the role play, the therapist can write on the board the list of assertiveness skills that may be used to deal with authority figures:

> Make eye contact and use appropriate body language.
> Listen attentively to what the person has to say.
> Apologize if needed.
> Offer a suggestion to avoid the problem in the future.

2.2. *Role-play the social skills relevant to preventing or solving conflict situations with adults.* The therapist should use modeling, corrective feedback, and reinforcement of appropriate social skills during this activity. If the child has difficulty engaging in a role play of real-life situations, use the hypothetical situations provided below.

- *Situation 1.* You arrive late for class because you were talking to your friend.
    TEACHER: You're late for class and I expect you to be here on time!
    You say . . .
- *Situation 2.* A teacher catches you passing a note to another student during class.
    TEACHER: You know that such behavior is not allowed in my classroom!
    You say . . .
- *Situation 3.* You did all your homework and are ready to go play with your friends, but your parent reminds you of a failed test and makes you stay home to study.
    PARENT: You better study some more so you don't fail any more tests!
    You say . . .
- *Situation 4.* Your parents ground you because of fighting with your little brother or sister.
    PARENT: Your sister is crying again. That's it. You are grounded for a month!
    You say . . .

Give as many opportunities as time permits to practice the four assertiveness skills listed in Section 2.1.

3. ***Discuss situations that lead to conflicts at home.*** The therapist could use the **Home Situations Questionnaire** to identify several situations that frequently lead to noncompliance at home. Parents can be told that this session is dedicated to developing a problem-solving strategy for one of these problem areas and that, as homework, their child will have to use this strategy at home. Some likely candidates for problems areas are:

> Fighting with a sibling.
> Not doing chores.
> Talking back or swearing at parents.

Your mom told me that there are a few things that you and she often argue about. Maybe you and I can develop a plan for solving one of these problems and you and your mom can agree on this plan at the end of the session.

Let's say the parents always argue with their daughter about the clothes she wears. The following is a discussion that took place with one of our patients:

THERAPIST: It looks like your mother is not always happy with the clothes you wear. She also said that you hate everything she buys for you and that you wear the same pair of old jeans all the time.

CHILD: I don't care what she thinks. That's what everyone wears.

THERAPIST: I hear that. So you say that you don't care what she thinks?

CHILD: Well, I don't care what she thinks about my clothes. I care what she thinks about other things.

THERAPIST: Like what?

CHILD: I know that she cares for me and all.

THERAPIST: So, it doesn't sound as if she bugs you about clothes just to annoy you. Why do you think she wants you to wear something else?

CHILD: I wear what I want to wear.

THERAPIST: So do I. But sometimes people still tell me what to wear, maybe not in so many words as your mom tells you.

CHILD: What do you mean?

THERAPIST: When I go hiking I wear hiking shoes, when I go to a Halloween party I wear a costume, and when I go to work I wear a tie. You sort of dress up for the occasion.

CHILD: Yeah, that's right. What's your point?

THERAPIST: Do you know why your mother is concerned about what you wear?

CHILD: She just ends up screaming at me when we talk about clothing. I am not gonna explain to her what people wear these days.

THERAPIST: People have very different fashion senses these days.

CHILD: Exactly.

THERAPIST: So by now we have spoken a lot about negotiating and problem solving. Can you use this knowledge to talk to your mom about clothes? It might make her happy.

CHILD: I can give it a try, what should I do?

THERAPIST: I'd like you to talk to your mom about it and figure out some compromise that you can both agree on. For example, you wear what she wants you to wear when you go to church on Sunday, and then you wear what you want to wear when you go to school on Monday.

CHILD: Well, what's in it for me? What you said is exactly what she wants me to do anyway.

THERAPIST: What's in it for you? Well, you'd make your mom very happy. You can't put a price tag on this. Also, if she is happy with what you wear maybe she will take you clothes shopping more often.

3.1. Using the **Home Situations Questionnaire,** the therapist should *review the list of common problem situations with the child as identified by the parent(s) and select the ones that the child agrees are common occurrences.* Therapists should be careful in using the **Home Situations Questionnaire** to avoid antagonizing the child with an unexpected revelation of his parents' opinions of their home life. If in doubt about the appropriateness of using the real parent report, just ask the child to provide his own examples of issues that cause frequent arguments at home.

Write down the relevant problem situations on a board or a piece of paper:

Home situation 1: _____

_____

Home situation 2: _____

_____

Home situation 3: _____

_____

Home situation 4: _____

_____

Discuss these situations using the following questions:

Why do you think this situation happens?
What do you do that makes your (mother, father, grandmother, etc.) angry at you?
What can you do to solve this problem if it happens again?

3.2. *Role-play finding a compromise for a real-life problem.* The therapist can use the **Home Situation Problem Solving** handout to describe the problem and the problem-solving strategy. Then the appropriate assertiveness skills, such as active listening and talking in a calm voice, can be role-played. Finally, the child can be asked to write down the plan for addressing this problem at home; the **Home Situation Problem Solving** handout provides a chart that can be filled out with the appropriate steps. A **Behavioral Contract** can be filled out where, if the child is successful in using the proposed strategy, the parents will provide a reasonable reward.

4. *Practice monitoring poor communication habits.* Use the **Communication Habits** handout and ask the child if he might have any of the communication habits that are listed on the left side of the handout. Clearly, the level of insight that children may have into their communication problems will vary considerably. However, everyone should be able to identify at least one or two habits that are less than helpful in conflict situations. It is also likely that the child's perception of his poor communication habits may be less dramatic than that of his parents. For example, the parents may be very concerned that their son uses foul language, while the child himself may have no awareness that he uses it.

Here is a list of poor communication habits. These are things that we do that may be annoying to others when we talk to them. Some of the habits, such as picking your nose in public, may be more obvious than others. For example, getting defensive is a common communication problem that people are often unaware of. Let's say your mom says, "Where is the remote?" and you say, "I didn't take it!" That exchange would be an example of getting defensive. Do you see how? [Have a brief discussion.] Let's go over this list to see if you recognize any of these communication habits in the way in which you talk with your mom.

4.1.   Provide the child with an index card to write down two or three poor communication habits he is both aware of and willing to work on.

So these are the poor habits that you've observed about yourself. What can you do or say instead of these habits? Would you say that the strategies listed on the right-hand side of the handout might work for you? Let's write down the good habits that you can use instead of the bad habits.

Bad communication habits can be discontinued (i.e., the person does nothing instead of engaging in habitual behavior) or replaced (i.e., the person engages in alternative behaviors). With communication habits, it is important to be aware of one's behavior as it unfolds. In other words, one has to use self-monitoring and catch the habit before it pops up again. The key to extinguishing a habitual behavior is to put oneself in a situation that would normally trigger the habit and then practice an alternative behavior.

I'd like for you to carry this index card around and look for some opportunities to practice good communication habits. For example, let's say you and your mom are about to take on a topic that might lead to an argument, such as homework, your curfew, etc. When you realize that you are about to get into a conversation that might provoke some of the poor communication habits we've discussed, take out this index card and keep it in front of you. [Model some unobtrusive way of looking at an index card and talking at the same time.] Then try to build the entire conversation on the positive communication habits listed on the card. I will also tell your mom to ease up on her requests when she sees you using this card.

To facilitate this exercise at home, the parents can be told about this assignment and asked to try "catching their child being good." The therapist can say to the parents that one of the homework assignments is to practice positive communication habits that are listed on the index card. If the parents see their son looking at this card, this is also a cue for them, showing them that he is trying to practice new good communication habits. This would be a good time for the parents to reciprocate their child's efforts and maybe make an extra step to find a compromise for the problem at hand.

5. ***Practice explaining one's role in a conflict situation.*** The goal of this activity is to teach the child to focus on the relevant points when discussing a problem. In a way, this is a summary of many skills that were covered before in the problem-solving and assertiveness skills sections. In this activity, the child should be prompted to focus on what's important in a conflict situation. Specifically, when there is a problem and an adult (parent or teacher) asks what happened, children don't always have the skills to clearly explain what happened. To develop this skill, the therapist should ask the child to go over one or two conflict situations and model how to communicate about what happened clearly.

One of the main goals of this program is to give you skills for dealing with problems. You have told me about several conflict situations, and we have worked together to come up with ways to help you solve these problems. [Give an example of one of the conflict situations reported by the child in previous sessions.] But telling about a problem clearly is also a strategy you can use to help solve the problem. If you don't describe and explain what happened clearly, this might complicate the solution. If a problem involves you directly, chances are you'll have to describe your role in a situation. Let's say you got into a fight in school and were sent to the principal's office. The principal will hear your side of the story and then the other guy's side of the story. Then the principal will make a ruling on who's right and who's wrong. The way you explain what happened may affect this decision.

Take a moment to discuss if the child appreciates the importance of clarity when advocating for oneself. To make a point more vivid, use several examples of when the child was able to explain what happened in a particular conflict clearly and when he might have given too little information or too many irrelevant details.

5.1. *Provide examples of poor storytelling.* One participant of the program came to his session and reported that he got suspended from school. When asked what happened, he said, "Because of this jerk teacher, he sent me to the principal." The whole story sounded like this:

This teacher always gets on my case. Even if I just sit and listen, he will find something wrong with that. And then, if someone else does something, he'll pay no attention to it. So there were these girls who were talking in class, and he said nothing to them. Then when I turned around to tell them to shut up, he sent me to the principal and I got suspended.

Ask the child if he thinks this story could be told in a better way.

The following conversation unfolded between the therapist and the patient to clarify the situation that led to school suspension.

THERAPIST: OK, is there more to it? Usually people don't get suspended for shushing someone.

CHILD: When I yelled at these girls so that they'd stop talking, I said I'd kill 'em. Of course, I didn't mean it, it's just a figure of speech.

THERAPIST: Well, you know these days, you can't say "I'd kill 'em" in school. It's like saying that you have a bomb on an airplane. It sounds as if you might have actually been suspended for making a "death threat" to these girls. Is that true?

CHILD: That's exactly how they twisted it.

THERAPIST: I think one of the reasons they twisted it like that is because you did not do a very good job telling your side of the story in the principal's office. If what you told there sounded like what you told me, they might have been left with an impression that you are an angry young man who also may be dangerous.

CHILD: I guess so.

THERAPIST: Let's try to use this situation to work on your skills to advocate for yourself. First of all, when something like that happens, you have to tell the story objectively. This means just describing what happened without exaggeration. Then, remember that a story should have a beginning, a middle, and an end. Unless you purposefully did something horrendous, the end of the story should have been that what happened was an unfortunate accident and you did everything you could to prevent it.

CHILD: OK.

THERAPIST: So let's start from the beginning. You said that you were suspended because the teacher was a jerk. That's not a winning line because when you blame people you also create an image of yourself as a hostile person. You want to give your listener an impression that you are a big-hearted, kind person. Can you think of a new opening line to your story?

CHILD: I think I know one. I was sitting and trying to focus on the lecture.

THERAPIST: That's excellent. It sends a message that you are in school to learn, that you are a motivated student. What's next?

CHILD: And these girls behind me were talking.

THERAPIST: I think this is a little too soon to bring up your classmates. You see, the truth is that you overreacted. It seems a little out of proportion to say "I'll kill you" if someone is just disrupting your concentration by talking.

CHILD: Well, they were talking for a long time and really annoying me.

THERAPIST: OK, but you need to set up a situation so that it will explain your behavior. For example, did you ask them nicely to stop talking? Were they doing anything other than just talking, such as saying something mean about you? Or throwing spit-balls at you?

CHILD: Yeah, they were laughing at me.

THERAPIST: You see, now the important details of the story are coming out. It sounds as if they were talking behind your back, laughing at you, and thus distracting you from paying attention in class. First, you tried to give them a half head-turn, like in the movies, hoping they'd stop. But they ignored you and continued talking.

CHILD: Yeah, and the teacher said nothing to them, but lashed out at me.

THERAPIST: I understand how in your view the teacher is an important part of this story. But if you take the outsider's perspective, like the principal's perspective, this situation mostly pertains to you and these girls. You see, even if you got angry because the teacher was unfair, you are better off sticking with the facts that other people also witnessed.

CHILD: So what do you want me to say?

THERAPIST: How about just saying how you feel. Remember the "I" statement approach?

CHILD: Well, I started to feel really angry.

THERAPIST: And when you started to feel angry, did you try to use any anger control techniques?

CHILD: Yeah, first I tried to ignore it, then I tried to take a few deep breaths, and then I just blew up.

THERAPIST: It looks like now you have a story that you could have told in the principal's office. How about something like this: "I was listening to Mr. Smith's lecture, trying to take notes. Then these noises and whispers started behind my back. It was two girls from my class, Jessica and Susan. After a few minutes I tried to look their way, hoping they'd stop talking. Probably because we all sit in the back of the classroom, Mr. Smith could not hear them, but for me it was really distracting. I tried to ignore this situation, but it was starting to make me angry. Then I tried to take a few deep breaths, but unfortunately my anger got the best of me by the middle of the class period. Clearly, I overreacted and I am sorry that I could not find a better way to handle the situation."

CHILD: That's exactly what happened.

THERAPIST: Another good thing to learn from this situation is that you should be careful about using threatening language.

5.2. Next, the therapist can *provide feedback to the child regarding his strengths and weaknesses in presenting his side of the story.* Ask the child to practice telling about conflict situations in short, direct sentences. The therapist should provide modeling and corrective feedback as the child formulates his thoughts. Here are some of the potential weakness areas:

Talking too much and not getting to the point:

People get confused and annoyed.

Blaming other people or being defensive:

You are perceived as hostile.

Missing important parts of the story:

The listener may have a distorted impression.

Not paying attention to the listener's feedback:

The listener may perceive you as rude.

Discuss the importance of following these rules:

Briefly describe the circumstances.
Don't blame other people.
Say how you felt, using "I" statements.
Focus on the main points; don't lose track of the presentation.
If you did something wrong, say that you are sorry.

6. ***Summarize the session and assign homework.*** Ask the child to recall the main points of the session and discuss how the material may be relevant to his current anger-provoking situations. A brief summary can be offered:

Today we spoke about problem-solving skills for conflicts with adults. We discussed some of the common situations that you may argue about with your parents at home. It looks like we have developed a plan for bringing one of these problem situations to an end. I hope you can stick with the plan and work on this situation at home. Then we also practiced the skill of clearly explaining one's role in a conflict situation.

6.1. *Ask the child to hold onto the index card with the communication habits and their alternative behaviors.* At the end of the session, remind the child to use these alternative behaviors at home and at school.

6.2. **Anger Management Log 9** should be filled out for the next session, describing one situation in which the child is able to successfully use any of the skills covered in this session.

6.3. At the end of the ninth session the **Daily Anger Monitoring Log** should be assigned again. The therapist should ask the child to record and briefly describe all incidents of anger that occur before the next session. The therapist and child should review the purpose of the **Daily Anger Monitoring Log** and discuss its categories. It should be emphasized that all anger-provoking events should be recorded.

7. ***Check in with parent(s).*** Ask the child to tell parents what he learned in session. Because this session is focused on parent–child conflict, this parent check-in may be somewhat longer than the others. The therapist can ask the child to summarize the content of the **Home Situation Problem Solving** handout for the parent. The parent may be asked to provide positive feedback on the child's description of the problem and his offered solution. If the child is interested in developing a **Behavioral Contract** (see Section 3.2 of this session), the therapist can help the child and his parent agree on the behavioral goals and rewards. Ask the parent to give an example of a time when their child was able to engage in appropriate behavior in a situation that could have triggered anger or noncompliance. If needed, therapists may provide two or three bullet points from the session material that resonated most with the child.

Review and Conclusion

★ GOALS

1. Collect homework and review the previous session's material.
2. Obtain the child's feedback on program effectiveness.
3. Conduct additional program review procedures.
4. Present the graduation diploma.
5. Check in with parent(s).

HANDOUTS

Disruptive Behavior Rating Scale

Home Situations Questionnaire

Checklist of Anger Management Skills

Graduation Diploma (optional)

HOMEWORK

None

1. *Collect homework and review the previous session's material.*

Last time we talked about dealing with conflict situations that involve parents and teachers. Sometimes these conflicts stem from misunderstandings or from acting without thinking. Then we spoke about assertiveness skills, including appropriate nonverbal behavior (body language, tone of voice, etc.) and active listening. These skills are particularly important in conflict negotiations with adults because nonverbal behavior can sometimes be misinterpreted by the adults as signs of disrespect. For example, you may think that if you raise your voice, it will increase your chances of being heard. Your mother, however, may think that raising your voice to her is disrespectful and she may get angry. Were you able to apply these assertiveness skills in any of the conflict situations during this past week?

We also practiced telling your side of the story in such a way that your actions are presented in a good light. Were there any situations during the past week that required you to use this skill?

1.1. *Review Anger Management Log 9.* If the child did not use assertive coping strategies, provide corrective feedback and model a more appropriate line of acting.

1.2. *Review the Daily Anger Monitoring Log* and ask if the child has included all significant anger episodes of the past week. Several minutes can be taken to discuss anger episodes reported in the log.

2. ***Obtain the child's feedback on program effectiveness.*** This part of the final session can be conducted as an interview and, if the child engages enough, this section can be extended into the bulk of the session. Below is a list of questions that can be used to guide this interview.

What did you think about the program in general? Has it been helpful?

We started with talking about anger, and I am curious to know if you have observed any differences in your anger experiences. Would you say that you get angry less often now than before, at the beginning of the program?

Would it be fair to say that there are fewer things that make you angry now than in the beginning? How about the intensity of your anger feelings? If something makes you angry now, does you anger rise to the extreme levels that it did before, or can you now keep it at a moderate level?

The therapist can rate the child's progress using the **Checklist of Anger Management Skills**. Parents can be asked to fill out the **Disruptive Behavior Rating Scale** and **Home Situations Questionnaire** for comparison with the baseline evaluation.

Summarize and highlight the positive changes reported by the child. For example:

It seems like you are less bothered by minor problems than you used to be.

2.1. *Review the anger management module of the program.* Ask the child to provide feedback on particular anger control skills that he has been able to use in his daily life. Clearly, by the end of the program, the therapist should have a pretty good idea about what the child has learned. Prompting might be used to facilitate the child's recall. The **Checklist of Anger Management Skills** contains a list of 10 techniques that were covered in the first three sessions. The therapist can either simply check off the techniques that the child has been using or, in a more fine-grained way, rank the techniques in order of their helpfulness as perceived by the child. The therapist may also rate the frequency with which the child has practiced these techniques.

Now let's think back about various anger management skills that we discussed in the program. What are the techniques that have been most helpful to you? How often do you use them?

Summarize the child's response and highlight the importance of practicing these skills on a continuous basis. For example:

It looks like you have been able to use a few strategies to manage your anger. You have been able to ignore small things and use reminders, like saying "Take it easy" to yourself. If you are having a bad day and frustrations seem to be piling up, you have also learned to take a time-out and listen to your favorite music. These are wonderful skills to have. The key is to continue using them for anger control even when our program is over.

If the therapist believes that the child has been using some skill but forgot to mention it in his review, it is appropriate to ask about this skill. However, therapists should avoid using this time to review something that has been forgotten or never used.

2.2. *Review the problem-solving module of the program.* Cognitive deficits in social problem solving are usually divided into cognitive deficiencies (i.e., lack of ability) and cognitive distortions (i.e., inadequate performance). The problem-solving module contained activities that target the child's deficiencies in generating, evaluating, and enacting appropriate conflict resolution strategies. In addition, there is a cognitive restructuring component that targets cognitive distortions in evaluating the significance of the provocation, understanding the other person's intentions, and legitimizing one's own aggressive behavior. The therapist should ask the child about any cognitive coping or problem-solving skills that he has been using in his day-to-day life. Check off or rate the techniques used by the child in the **Checklist of Anger Management Skills.**

We've spent some time talking about thinking before acting, generating several solutions to a problem, and thinking about the consequences of our behavior. Have these suggestions been helpful to you in dealing with problem situations? We've also spent some time learning to better understand the causes of conflict situations and other people's motivations in them. Have you been able to use this information in your life?

Summarize the child's response to one or two of the problem-solving strategies that have worked best for him, and highlight the importance of continuing to practice these strategies. For example:

So you are saying that it has been helpful for you to think about the different ways in which you can solve a problem before you actually do anything. This approach gives you more choices. You also have been trying to put yourself into another person's shoes to understand the causes of his actions. If you do that and you realize the problem wasn't really his fault, but was actually an accident, you will be less likely to get angry.

Again, if the therapist believes that the child uses more problem-solving skills than he mentioned in this review, it is appropriate to do further probing. However, therapists should not use this time to go over the forgotten, and therefore irrelevant material.

2.3. *Review the social skills training module of the program.* The goal of this component was to develop appropriate skills for dealing with peer and adult conflict situations. These social skills consisted of various assertiveness techniques, such as active listening, modulating one's nonverbal behavior, and offering an explanation of one's behavior in a problem situation. Similar to the review of the two previous modules, ask the child if he has been able to use any of the social skills and assertiveness techniques.

In the last three sessions of our program we practiced various skills that could be helpful in resolving conflict situations. The most important part was learning to use words to solve problems. Do you think it has been easier for you to communicate and negotiate conflict situations after what we've done in the program?
We also spoke about body language, facial expressions, and vocal qualities. These are all part of the package called assertive behavior. Acting assertively means doing something to straighten out a problem without offending the other people involved. Were you able to use any of the assertiveness techniques at home or in school?

Summarize the child's response to the questions about the social skills training and highlight the importance of using those skills that have already been helpful on a continuous basis. For example:

It sounds like you have learned not to raise your voice when you talk to your mother and to focus on the relevant details when explaining your behavior to someone in authority. You have also said that learning to listen carefully to another person when you have an argument with him or her has improved your communication with both your parents and your teachers.

If the child did not offer any detailed feedback, it is OK to probe with more specific questions. However, the therapist should be careful not to lecture or talk about something that has not worked before.

3. ***Conduct additional program review procedures.*** There are several alternative ways to review the program. These include comparing **Daily Anger Monitoring Logs** from the beginning and the end of the program, and reviewing the child's feedback to each session for a simplified version of the review. The therapist may choose from these activities depending on the child's overall progress in the program.

3.1. *Compare **Daily Anger Monitoring Logs** from the beginning and the end of the program.* To prepare for this activity, the therapist must have the **Daily Anger Monitoring Logs** from the first two sessions. In this treatment, **Anger Monitoring Logs** are used for their clinical value, that is, to teach self-monitoring, rather than for their psychometric value. The therapist may first review the logs and prepare the feedback for the child. This feedback can focus on comparing the child's self-reports of frequency, intensity, and duration of anger episodes at the beginning and at the end of the program.

3.2. *Review the child's feedback to each session.* Each session ended with the therapist asking the child about the relevant and feasible coping mechanisms discussed during that session. Then, each following session started with the therapist asking the child about how these coping mechanisms worked during the week. Consequently, the last session's review can be focused on those skills that have been noted by the child during reviews of each session's homework.

4. ***Present the Graduation Diploma.*** Many of the children whom we worked with participated in this treatment as part of clinical research. We found that younger children (8- to 12-year-olds) enjoyed receiving what we call a **Graduation Diploma**. Therapists may use their clinical judgment to decide whether to issue a graduation diploma or to just go with a handshake and a "thank you" as a way to conclude the last session of this treatment. Some families may ask for booster sessions, which can be provided as needed and consist of rehearsing anger management and problem-solving skills that resonated the most with the child.

5. ***Check in with parent(s).*** At the end of the last session, parents could be invited for a longer visit in order to obtain feedback, review progress, and conclude the program.

PARENT SESSIONS

Even though CBT is a child-focused treatment, it would be clinically counter-productive and unnatural for the therapists to have no contact with the parents. In our clinical studies we had three 30-minute parent sessions that were scheduled either before or after child sessions in the beginning, middle, and at the end of the treatment. In clinical practice, parent sessions could be scheduled as collateral visits on an as-needed basis. The therapists should also conduct brief check-ins with the parents in order to summarize the content of each session and allow the parents an opportunity to acknowledge their child's work in the program.

Most common forms of disruptive behavior occur in families and include noncompliance with parental requests, arguing, and sibling conflict. As part of CBT, children will be taught problem-solving skills and alternative behaviors to prevent these problems. Parents should provide praise and rewards for their children's appropriate behavior. We note in the Introduction that various parent training programs are available to help parents learn strategies for dealing with child's disruptive behavior. As part of this child-focused CBT, therapists may provide parents with education about the value of reinforcement in shaping their child's maladaptive as well as positive behavior. We encourage parents to pay attention and praise children for not misbehaving or, using the words of Russell Barkley, "catch them being good" (Barkley, 1997). We usually also ask parents to model for their children appropriate anger management skills such as using a calm tone of voice when discussing frustrating situations.

Parent Session 1

The first meeting with the parents is similar to the first encounter in psychotherapy. Ideally, it should take place right before the first child session.

★ GOALS

1. Welcome parents to the program.
2. Gather information.
3. Provide information about the purpose, format, and content of CBT.
4. Educate parents about praising and rewarding desirable behavior.

HANDOUTS

Disruptive Behavior Rating Scale (DBRS) (for parents)

Home Situations Questionnaire (HSQ) (for parents)

1. ***Welcome parents to the program.*** Therapists can start by providing a general welcome to the program by inquiring about the presenting complaints and describing the format of the treatment. Therapists may also ask the parent to complete the **Home Situations Questionnaire** and the **Disruptive Behavior Rating Scale** before the first session to evaluate the child's current levels of anger and noncompliance. The total scores can also provide helpful information about the overall seriousness of behavioral problems. Responses to the individual items may provide helpful clinical information about the frequency and types of disruptive behavior.

Some topics, such as scheduling and goals about reducing behaviors like fighting, can be addressed with the parent and child together at the beginning of the program.

> I'd like to take a few moments to review this treatment. There will be 10 weekly sessions. Most of the time they will be conducted one-on-one with the child. Sometimes we will meet as a group and sometimes I will catch up one-on-one with the parents. What are your expectations for this program?

2. *Gather information.* The child can be asked to wait outside while relevant information collected during the child's clinical evaluation is reviewed and discussed. The therapist should focus on the behavioral problems that can be targeted with this treatment, and explain to the parents how CBT will address these symptoms. Therapists who were not involved in the initial clinical evaluation should familiarize themselves with the information that has been collected. This might be the case in clinics where intake evaluation is conducted by one clinician who then assigns the child to a therapist, or in research studies where evaluation and therapy are also conducted by different individuals. Therapists who have conducted an evaluation of the child themselves may review the findings with the parents at this time.

The following areas are particularly important to review:

Particular behavioral problems and their severity.
Times and situations when the problems are most likely to occur.
How these problems have been addressed so far.
History of treatment.
Current family stressors.
Any psychiatric diagnosis and symptoms other than disruptive behavior.

3. *Provide information about the purpose, format, and content of CBT.* This can be done when the child is in the room, but the review can be geared to the adult level.

> This cognitive-behavioral therapy—CBT—teaches emotion regulation and problem solving. The goal of this CBT treatment is to reduce the frequency and intensity of anger or related disruptive behaviors.
>
> Do you have any questions about this program?

It is important to discuss scheduling and to address issues such as missed sessions, rescheduling, being late, parking, and the like. It should be also mentioned that CBT involves practicing certain skills at home ("homework" could be a bad word to use in front of the child) but this is not like homework at school, and the parents should not demand anything from their child. Throughout the treatment, therapists should strive to have the child "own" the program and be responsible for carrying out assignments for practicing anger management skills at home.

4. ***Educate parents about praising and rewarding desirable behavior.*** Parents should be informed about the importance of praising and rewarding their child for engaging in desirable behaviors and also for not engaging in disruptive behaviors. "Catch them being good" is a helpful way to convey to the parents the importance of giving attention and praise to children when they are not misbehaving. It may also be helpful if parents provide rewards for attending CBT, which may include praise for the effort as well as tangible reinforcements such as stopping on the way home for a treat after the session.

Similarly, parents can be advised to ignore minor misbehaviors and learn to "pick their fights" in order to avoid inadvertently reinforcing their child's misbehavior by letting him win (a mechanism known as "escape conditioning"). For example, a driver is likely to slow down after getting a speeding ticket, and a child is likely to have another tantrum if previous tantrums have led to getting his way. Behaviors such as noncompliance, whining, or bickering can be reinforced if they result in escape or avoidance of situations such as homework or room cleaning, which could be aversive to the child.

Positive reinforcement of desirable behavior, such as doing homework or sharing the TV remote with siblings, is at the core of behavioral management. Although intuitively appealing, reinforcement principles and techniques may be misinterpreted. For example, when social reinforcement such as attention and praise is discussed with parents, a common reaction is, "We do it all the time." However, further discussions often reveal that attention may be given to disruptive behavior while appropriate behavior may go unrecognized by praise.

Detailed discussion of punishment may be outside the scope of this program, but it can be noted that punishment alone is unlikely to change behavior. Harsh and inconsistent discipline such as excessive verbal scolding and corporal punishment has been shown to increase aggression.

Parent Session 2

The second 30-minute meeting can be conducted before or after the fifth child session, at the midpoint of the treatment.

★ GOALS

1. Discuss the child's progress in the program.
2. Provide the parent with feedback about the child's interest in the program and report some intermediate results.
3. Emphasize that improvement may take more time.
4. Find out about the ongoing and/or new events that may be relevant to the treatment.
5. Coordinate treatment with other adults invested in the child's success.

1. ***Discuss the child's progress in the program.*** Ask about any changes in the level of the targeted disruptive behavior symptoms, new problem areas, and new stressors or relevant events.

Do you see any improvement in behavior?
Have any new problems arisen?
How does he like treatment so far?
Have you seen him use any anger management skills at home?

2. **_Provide the parent with feedback about the child's interest in the program and report some intermediate results._** For example:

He has been motivated and interested in the program.
He tells me that he has been able to apply some of the anger management skills, such as thinking about consequences before acting in conflict situations.

3. **_Emphasize that improvement may take more time,_** if the parents say that there is no improvement or report new behavioral problems. Discuss the lack of progress and encourage the family to continue CBT.

Behavioral change is gradual, and it might take more time for the improvements to show. Can you remember any instances of appropriate behavior in place of what could have been an argument or an instance of noncompliance?

4. **_Find out about the ongoing and/or new events that may be relevant to the treatment._** For example, if the family is going through a divorce, the possible impact of this event on the child's disruptive behavior may need to be explored. If the parent reports a new stressor, such as illness of a family member or financial problems, psychological support should be provided as clinically relevant. Some of the guiding questions for this area are as follows:

How are things at home? Is everyone doing well?
If there is a new stressor, how is the child responding to it?

5. **_Coordinate treatment with other adults invested in the child's success._** It is not uncommon for parents of children who participate in CBT for anger and aggression to request that information about their child's participation in this study be shared with their child's teachers or principal, or other clinicians. The therapist should remember to have the parents sign consent forms allowing for the release or exchange of information prior to issuing any letters or reports about their clients.

Parent Session 3

The third parent session should be conducted at the end of the treatment, either before or after the final child session, in order to obtain feedback, review progress, and conclude the program.

★ GOALS

1. Discuss the child's progress.
2. Review any changes in targeted behavioral problems.
3. Conclude treatment.

1. ***Discuss the child's progress.*** Obtain the parents' feedback about anger management skills that the child has been able to use at home, review the change in frequency and intensity of target behaviors since the beginning of the program, and ask the parents what they think about the program in general (informal consumer satisfaction survey).

So what do you think about this treatment?

Would you recommend it to someone else?

Were you able to observe your child using some of the anger management skills that were part of the treatment?

2.   ***Review any changes in targeted behavioral problems.*** Provide education about other treatments for persistent behavioral problems (see Introduction for details).

Let's recall some of the behavioral problems that you noted in the beginning of the treatment. What is the frequency of these behaviors now?

Some other treatments for persistent behavioral problems include structured parent management training, multicomponential treatments such as multisystemic therapy (MST), and medication management.

3.   ***Conclude treatment.*** Thank the parents for participation in the treatment. Suggest clinical resources if needed.

APPENDIX 1

CLIENT HANDOUTS

Elements of an Anger Episode

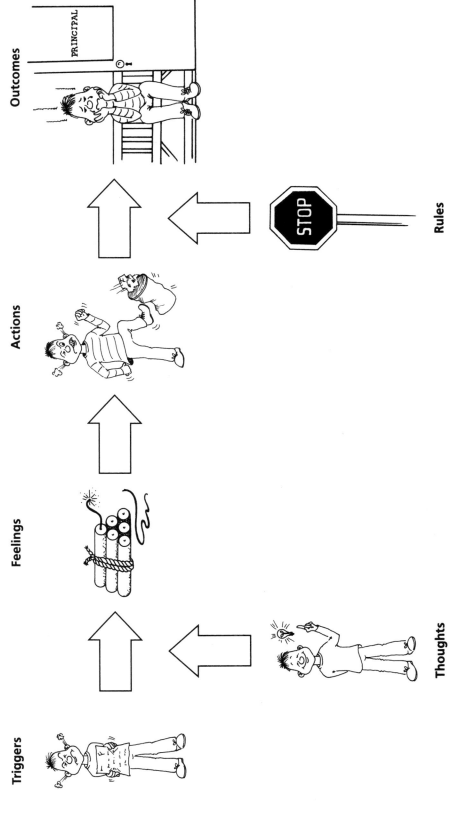

Triggers **Feelings** **Actions** **Outcomes**

Thoughts **Rules**

PRINCIPAL

STOP

Anger Triggers

Common Anger Triggers	**Your Anger Triggers**
	1. _____
	2. _____
	3. _____
	4. _____
	5. _____

Distract Yourself from Anger

Things people do to distract from anger:

What can you do to distract yourself when you're angry?

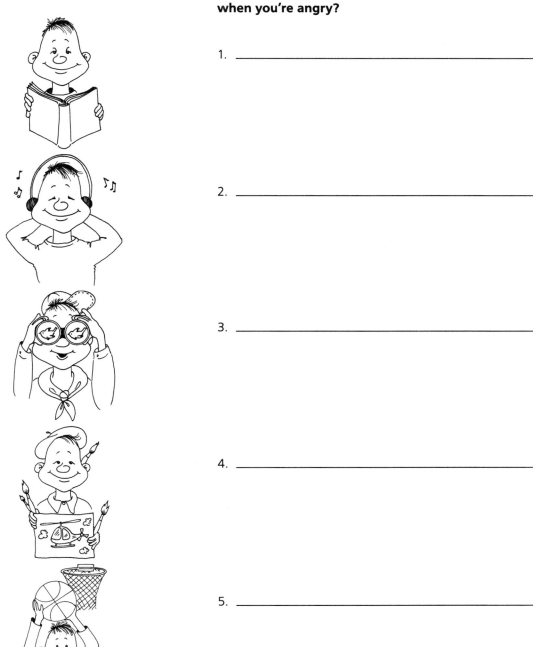

1. _____

2. _____

3. _____

4. _____

5. _____

HANDOUT 4

Daily Anger Monitoring Log

Instructions: Describe all anger-provoking situations that happen to you during the week between sessions. Try to take a few minutes by the end of each day to describe the events of this day. Don't put off filling out this chart to the last moment before it is due. It is very important that you monitor events that make you angry on a daily basis. If you run out of space, continue on reverse.

Date/time/place	What made you angry?	Anger intensity (0–100)	What did you do?	Consequences?
1.				
2.				
3.				
4.				
5.				
6.				
7.				

(cont.)

Daily Anger Monitoring Log *(page 2 of 2)*

Date/time/place	What made you angry?	Anger intensity (0–100)	What did you do?	Consequences?
8.				
9.				
10.				
11.				
12.				
13.				
14.				

Don't forget to bring this with you to the next session!

Anger Management Log 1

Recall one situation during this week when something made you angry and you handled it well using the anger management skills.

Describe this situation: _____

_____

_____

Who was involved? _____

_____

_____

What did you say? _____

_____

_____

What did you do? _____

_____

_____

What happened after? _____

_____

_____

Is there anything that you could have done differently? _____

_____

_____

Day _____ Time _____ Location _____

Feeling Thermometer

Temp	Feeling	Control
—very hot	rage	_____
—hot	anger	_____
—mild	frustration	_____
—cool	annoyance	_____
—cold	discomfort	_____

Stop Sign

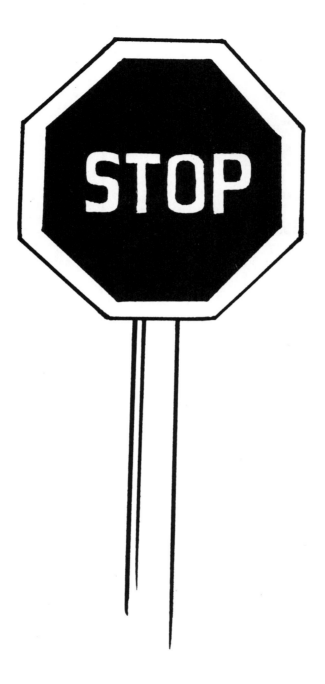

Words for Anger

Which of these words mean that a person feels less angry, and which of these words mean that a person feels very angry?

	VERY ANGRY	LESS ANGRY
Angry	_____	_____
Furious	_____	_____
Annoyed	_____	_____
Frustrated	_____	_____
Mad	_____	_____
Offended	_____	_____
Irritated	_____	_____
Sore	_____	_____
Grouchy	_____	_____
Mean	_____	_____
Upset	_____	_____
Sullen	_____	_____
Gloomy	_____	_____
Blew a fuse	_____	_____
Pain in the neck	_____	_____
On my nerves	_____	_____
Steamed	_____	_____
Burned up	_____	_____
Oscar the Grouch	_____	_____

Relaxation Practice Log 1

Try to use each of the relaxation strategies at least once a day. Write down the date, time, and location for each time you had a chance to use one of these techniques.

	Day	Time	Location
Rhythmic Breathing			
Positive Imagery			
Counting Backward			

	Day	Time	Location
Rhythmic Breathing			
Positive Imagery			
Counting Backward			

	Day	Time	Location
Rhythmic Breathing			
Positive Imagery			
Counting Backward			

	Day	Time	Location
Rhythmic Breathing			
Positive Imagery			
Counting Backward			

	Day	Time	Location
Rhythmic Breathing			
Positive Imagery			
Counting Backward			

Anger Management Log 2

Recall one situation during this week when something made you angry and you handled it well using the anger management skills.

Describe this situation: _____

_____

_____

How angry were you? _____

_____

_____

What reminders did you use to avoid getting in trouble? _____

_____

_____

What did you say? _____

_____

_____

What happened after? _____

_____

_____

Is there anything that you could have done differently in this situation? _____

_____

_____

Day _____ Time _____ Location _____

Where Do You Feel Anger Inside?

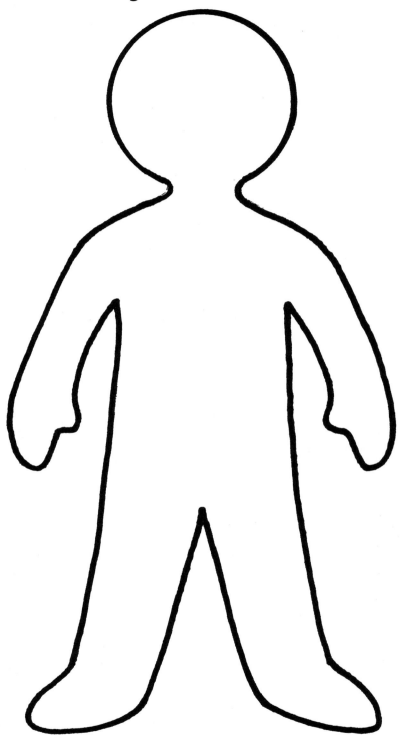

The Many Faces of Anger

What do people look like when they are angry?

_____

_____

_____

_____

_____

_____

_____

What do you look like when you are angry?

_____

_____

_____

_____

_____

_____

_____

_____

Drawing Anger

In the space below, draw whatever images come to your mind when you think about being angry.

Progressive Muscle Relaxation

Tense each muscle group for 5 seconds and then relax for 15 seconds.
Concentrate on slow, relaxing breathing while doing this exercise.

1. Clench both fists. ————————————————→ hands and forearms

2. Bend both elbows. ————————————————→ biceps

3. Frown and clench teeth. ——————————————→ face and jaw

4. Push head back and down. —————————————→ neck

5. Push shoulder blades together. ————————————→ shoulders and back

6. Tense stomach muscles. ——————————————→ abdominal region

7. Raise legs out, curling feet. —————————————→ thighs

8. Keep legs up, curl toes down. ————————————→ calves, feet, and toes

Anger Management Log 3

Describe a situation during this week when something made you angry and you handled it using the anger management skills.

Describe this situation: _____

_____

_____

Did you try to prevent the situation? _____

_____

Did you monitor the intensity of your anger? _____

_____

What did you do to feel less angry? _____

_____

Did you use relaxation techniques? _____

_____

How did this situation end? _____

_____

Is there anything that you could have done differently? _____

_____

_____

Day _____ Time _____ Location _____

Relaxation Practice Log 2

Try to use each of the relaxation strategies at least once a day. Write down the date, time, and location for every time you had a chance to use one of these techniques.

	Day	Time	Location
Rhythmic Breathing			
Positive Imagery			
Counting Backward			
Muscle Relaxation			

	Day	Time	Location
Rhythmic Breathing			
Positive Imagery			
Counting Backward			
Muscle Relaxation			

	Day	Time	Location
Rhythmic Breathing			
Positive Imagery			
Counting Backward			
Muscle Relaxation			

	Day	Time	Location
Rhythmic Breathing			
Positive Imagery			
Counting Backward			
Muscle Relaxation			

Calming Thoughts

Make a list of things that really make you angry. Then write down "calming thoughts." Calming thoughts are things you can think in your head to keep yourself from getting angry.

It makes me angry when someone:

_____

_____

I can calm down by thinking:

_____

_____

It makes me angry when someone:

_____

_____

I can calm down by thinking:

_____

_____

It makes me angry when someone:

_____

_____

I can calm down by thinking:

_____

_____

Blind Men and a Large Object

A group of blind men came across a large object and were trying to figure out what it was. Each of them placed a hand on the object and told the others what he felt. Here is a list of things they thought they felt, but none of them were correct.

Tree. What might feel like a tree that is not a tree? _____

_____

Rope. What might feel like a rope that is not a rope? _____

_____

Horn. What might feel like a horn that is not a horn? _____

_____

Wall. What might feel like a wall that is not a wall? _____

_____

Snake. What might feel like a snake that is not a snake? _____

_____

Fan. What might feel like a fan that is not a fan? _____

_____

Can you think of something that might feel like all of these things? _____

_____

Anger Management Log 4

Recall one situation during this week when something made you angry and you handled it well using the anger management skills.

What happened? _____

_____

Who was involved? _____

_____

What was the problem for you? _____

_____

What was the problem for the other person? _____

_____

Why did the other person do what he did? _____

_____

What are some *other possible reasons* for what he did? _____

_____

_____

What were your goals in this situation? _____

_____

What were the other person's goals? _____

_____

Day _____ Time _____ Location _____

Problem Identification, Choices, and Consequences (PICC)

I. *P*roblem *I*dentification

1. What was the problem? _____

2. What did you do? _____

3. What did the other person do? _____

II. *C*hoices

A. What could you have been done in the situation?

III. *C*onsequences (for each choice)

1. I could have _____   1. _____

2. I could have _____   2. _____

3. I could have _____   3. _____

B. What is the best choice (solution) to this problem? _____

_____

_____

_____

_____

Manage Anger before Problem Solving (MAPS)

How did I know that I was angry?

What was the situation? _____

Were there any signs of anger in my body? _____

What words ran through my head? _____

What did I do to manage my anger and to cool off?

Breathing, relaxation? _____

Calming self-talk? _____

Distraction? _____

Did I use problem-solving skills?

What were my choices? _____

_____

_____

What were the consequences? _____

_____

_____

What was the solution? _____

_____

_____

Words to Express Anger Politely

It is possible to express anger politely. You can use phrases such as:

Please stop it.

Don't do that.

I am angry because . . .

Knock it off.

Leave me alone.

I don't like that.

Cut it out.

Can you think of some more ideas?

_____   _____   _____

_____   _____   _____

_____   _____   _____

_____   _____   _____

_____   _____   _____

_____   _____   _____

_____   _____   _____

Anger Management Log 5

Recall one situation during this week when something made you angry and you handled it well using anger management skills.

What was the problem as you saw it? _____

What were your goal(s) in the situation? _____

What were the other person's goal(s) in the situation? _____

What choices did you have in this situation? _____

Alternative Solutions

A. I could have _____

B. I could have _____

C. I could have _____

What would have been the consequence to each of these alternative choices?

A. _____

B. _____

C. _____

What was the best solution and why? _____

_____

What did you *actually* do? (What choice did you make?) _____

_____

What happened after you made that choice?

_____

_____

Day _____   Time _____   Location _____

Fishing Boat

Imagine you are on a fishing boat that has run into bad weather and engine trouble several miles from shore. The captain has told you that because of the rough weather, the boat needs to be lighter to avoid sinking. You, as a member of the crew, need to decide which items to keep and which items to throw overboard. *You are only allowed to keep three items.*

List of items	What would you do?	
Matches	Keep	Throw overboard
Radio	Keep	Throw overboard
Compass	Keep	Throw overboard
Navigational map	Keep	Throw overboard
10 gallons of water	Keep	Throw overboard
Signal flares	Keep	Throw overboard
Life rafts	Keep	Throw overboard
Flashlight	Keep	Throw overboard
Life jackets	Keep	Throw overboard

Behavioral Contract

This contract between _____ and his/her parent(s) _____

With regard to the following:

1. _____

_____

2. _____

_____

It is agreed that _____ will do the following:

1. _____

_____

2. _____

_____

In return, _____ (parents) agree to:

1. _____

_____

2. _____

_____

All parties have read and discussed this agreement. Any exceptions must be mutually agreed upon by all parties. If disputes arise, changes to the contract may be negotiated in the future.

Signed by _____   _____

Date _____   _____

Anger Management Log 6

Recall one situation during this week when something made you angry and you handled it well using the anger management skills.

What was the problem? _____

_____

Did you think about the consequences? _____

Is there anything you would have done differently in this situation? _____

    (1) I could have _____

    (2) I could have _____

    (3) I could have _____

What would have been the consequences to these choices?

    (1) _____

    (2) _____

    (3) _____

What was the best solution? _____

_____

What did you *actually* do? _____

_____

Day _____ Time _____ Location _____

Role-Play Practice

Imagine that you are Mr. Smith, the teacher at the junior high school.

Your student (the therapist) does not pay attention in class.

You say: **"How many times have I told you to pay attention?"**

Listen carefully to what your therapist says.

How do you think the teacher would have responded?

Role-play his reaction.

Don't be afraid to get creative: think about body language and tone of voice, not just the words.

Three Ways of Acting

Passive. Doing nothing when something bad happens to you.

    (Ignoring)

What do you think about this way of acting?

_____

_____

_____

_____

Aggressive.   Fighting or yelling back when something happens to you.

    (Getting in trouble)

What do you think about this way of acting?

_____

_____

_____

_____

Assertive.   Talking the problem out and negotiating.

    (Achieving your goals)

What do you think about this way of acting?

_____

_____

_____

_____

Anger Management Log 7a
(Assertive Response to Teasing)

Who was teasing you? _____

What was this person saying? _____

What did you say in response? _____

Did you say it in a calm voice? _____ yes _____ no

Did you use any threatening gestures? _____ yes _____ no

Did you leave enough personal space? _____ yes _____ no

What happened afterward? _____

_____

_____

Is there anything that you could have done differently in this situation? _____

_____

_____

Day _____ Time _____ Location _____

Anger Management Log 7b
(Ignoring Teasing)

Who was teasing you? _____

What was this person saying? _____

_____

_____

What did you say in response? _____

_____

_____

Were you able to ignore the teasing? _____ yes _____ no

What happened afterward? _____

_____

_____

Is there anything that you could have done differently in this situation? _____

_____

_____

Day _____ Time _____ Location _____

The Bill of Rights

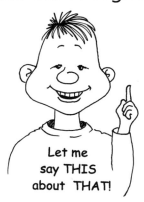

Let me
say THIS
about THAT!

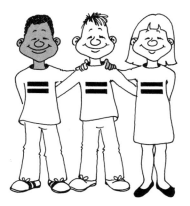

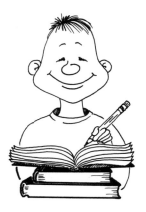

Three Steps of Active Listening

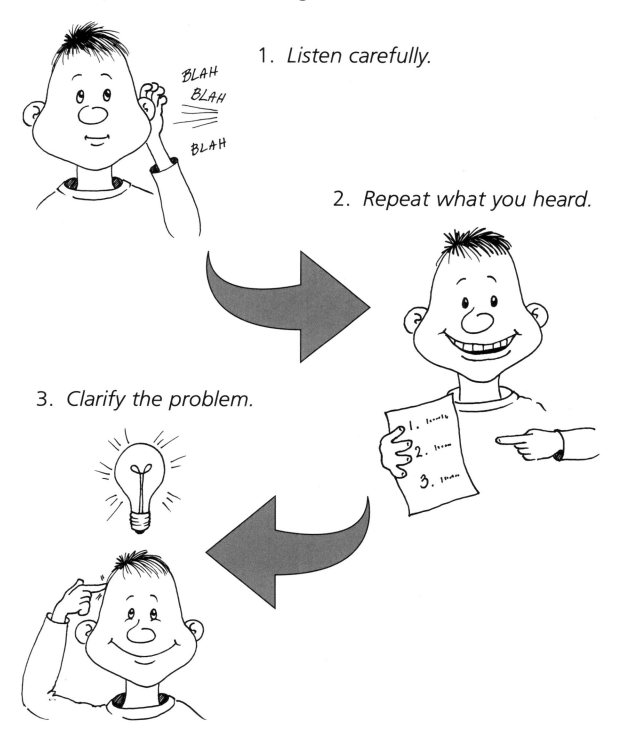

1. *Listen carefully.*

2. *Repeat what you heard.*

3. *Clarify the problem.*

Anger Management Log 8a
(Assertiveness Skills)

Describe the conflict: _____

_____

_____

What did you say? _____

_____

_____

Did you say it in a calm voice? _____ yes _____ no

Did you have a neutral facial expression? _____ yes _____ no

What happened afterward? _____

_____

_____

Is there anything that you could have done differently in this situation? _____

_____

_____

Day _____ Time _____ Location _____

Anger Management Log 8b
(Dealing with Accusation)

Describe the conflict: _____

_____

_____

Did you deserve the blame? _____

_____

_____

Were you able to listen first? _____ yes _____ no

How did you clarify the situation? _____

_____

_____

What did you say in the end? _____

_____

_____

Did you say it in a calm voice? _____ yes _____ no

Did you use any gestures? _____ yes _____ no

If yes, which ones? _____

What happened afterward? _____

_____

_____

Is there anything that you could have done differently in this situation? _____

_____

_____

Day _____ Time _____ Location _____

Home Situation Problem Solving

Describe a common conflict situation at home.

_____

_____

Why is this a problem for you?

_____

_____

_____

Why is this a problem for your parents?

_____

_____

_____

What is the best thing you can do to solve this problem?

_____

_____

_____

How can you communicate about this solution with your parents?

_____

_____

_____

What anger management skills can be used as you are implementing this solution?

_____

_____

_____

Communication Habits

Poor	Good
Insults	State the issue
Interrupts	Take turns
Criticizes	Note good and bad
Gets defensive	Calmly disagree
Lectures	Short and straight
Looks away	Make eye contact
Slouches	Sit up straight
Uses sarcasm	Talk in normal tone
Goes silent	Say what you feel
Denies	Accept responsibility
Commands, orders	Ask nicely
Yells	Use normal tone of voice
Swears	Use respectful language
Throws a tantrum	Cool it, count to 10

General Principles of Good Communication

1. Listen when the other person is in the mood to talk.
2. Use active listening.
3. Honestly express how you feel without being hurtful to your listener.

Anger Management Log 9
(Assertive Skills for Problem Solving with Adults)

Describe the situation: _____

_____

_____

_____

What did you say? _____

_____

_____

_____

Did you use a calm voice? _____ yes _____ no

Did you make eye contact? _____ yes _____ no

Did you listen carefully? _____ yes _____ no

Did you have to apologize? _____ yes _____ no

Did you offer a solution? _____ yes _____ no

How did the situation end? _____

_____

_____

_____

Day _____ Time _____ Location _____

Graduation Diploma

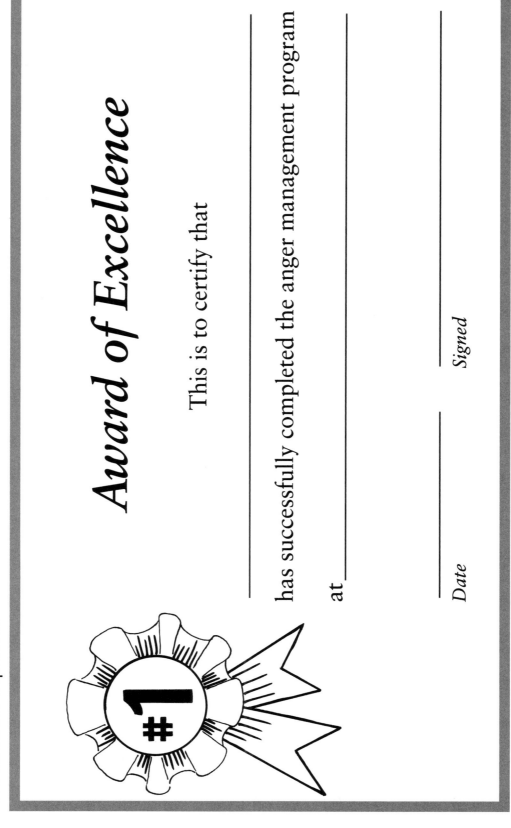

Award of Excellence

This is to certify that

_____

has successfully completed the anger management program

at _____

_____
Date

_____
Signed

Disruptive Behavior Rating Scale (DBRS)

Child's name _____ Date _____

Name of person completing this form _____

Relationship to child _____

Instructions: Please circle the number next to each item that best describes the behavior of this child <u>during the past week</u>.

	Never or rarely (once a week or less)	Sometimes (2–3 times a week)	Often (almost every day)	Very often (every day or several times a day)
1. Loses temper	0	1	2	3
2. Argues with adults	0	1	2	3
3. Actively defies or refuses to comply with adult's requests or rules	0	1	2	3
4. Deliberately annoys people	0	1	2	3
5. Blames others for his/her mistakes or misbehaviors	0	1	2	3
6. Is touchy or easily annoyed by others	0	1	2	3
7. Is angry or resentful	0	1	2	3
8. Is spiteful or vindictive	0	1	2	3

Total Score [ ]

Do these ratings reflect how things have been going lately (past month)?   Yes   No

Home Situations Questionnaire (HSQ)

Child's name _____ Date _____

Name of person completing this form _____

Relationship to child _____

Instructions: Does your child present any problems with compliance to instructions, commands, or rules for you in any of these situations? If so, please circle the word Yes and then circle a number beside that situation that describes how severe the problem is for you. If your child is not a problem in a situation, circle No and go on to the next situation on the form. If there are any situations that are problematic but they have not been mentioned on the list, please write them down in the provided space and rate their severity.

Situations	Yes/No	Mild								Severe
					If yes, how severe?					
1. While playing alone	Yes No	1	2	3	4	5	6	7	8	9
2. While playing with other children	Yes No	1	2	3	4	5	6	7	8	9
3. At mealtimes	Yes No	1	2	3	4	5	6	7	8	9
4. Getting dressed	Yes No	1	2	3	4	5	6	7	8	9
5. Washing and bathing	Yes No	1	2	3	4	5	6	7	8	9
6. While you are on the telephone	Yes No	1	2	3	4	5	6	7	8	9
7. While watching television	Yes No	1	2	3	4	5	6	7	8	9
8. When visitors are in your home	Yes No	1	2	3	4	5	6	7	8	9
9. When you are visiting someone's home	Yes No	1	2	3	4	5	6	7	8	9
10. In public places (restaurants, stores)	Yes No	1	2	3	4	5	6	7	8	9
11. When father is home	Yes No	1	2	3	4	5	6	7	8	9
12. When asked to do chores	Yes No	1	2	3	4	5	6	7	8	9
13. When asked to do homework	Yes No	1	2	3	4	5	6	7	8	9

(cont.)

Home Situations Questionnaire (HSQ) *(page 2 of 2)*

Situations	Yes/No	Mild				*If yes, how severe?*				Severe
14. At bedtime	Yes No	1	2	3	4	5	6	7	8	9
15. While in the car	Yes No	1	2	3	4	5	6	7	8	9
16. When with a babysitter	Yes No	1	2	3	4	5	6	7	8	9
17. Getting up in the morning	Yes No	1	2	3	4	5	6	7	8	9
18. Messing up the house	Yes No	1	2	3	4	5	6	7	8	9
19. Going to school on time	Yes No	1	2	3	4	5	6	7	8	9
20. Coming home on time	Yes No	1	2	3	4	5	6	7	8	9
21.	Yes No	1	2	3	4	5	6	7	8	9
22.	Yes No	1	2	3	4	5	6	7	8	9
23.	Yes No	1	2	3	4	5	6	7	8	9
24.	Yes No	1	2	3	4	5	6	7	8	9
25.	Yes No	1	2	3	4	5	6	7	8	9

Total number of problem settings _____ Mean severity score _____

Checklist of Anger Management Skills

Global Change in Frequency and Intensity of Anger:

Frequency of anger episodes	Much lower	Lower	Same	Higher
Number of anger triggers	Much lower	Lower	Same	Higher
Intensity of anger experiences	Much lower	Lower	Same	Higher

Anger Management Skills:

Ignoring the provocation	Always	Sometimes	Never
Distraction from the frustrating situation	Always	Sometimes	Never
Engaging in competing pleasant activities	Always	Sometimes	Never
Self-monitoring of anger arousal	Always	Sometimes	Never
The Stop and Think technique	Always	Sometimes	Never
Using reminders to cool off	Always	Sometimes	Never
Deep breathing	Always	Sometimes	Never
Counting backward	Always	Sometimes	Never
Positive imagery	Always	Sometimes	Never
Muscle relaxation	Always	Sometimes	Never

Problem-Solving Skills:

Thinking about why there is a problem	Always	Sometimes	Never
Thinking about consequences of actions	Always	Sometimes	Never
Considering another person's motives	Always	Sometimes	Never
Generating multiple solutions	Always	Sometimes	Never
Evaluating different types of consequences	Always	Sometimes	Never
Analyzing ambiguous causes	Always	Sometimes	Never
Reducing hostile attribution bias	Always	Sometimes	Never
Avoiding inflammatory anger words	Always	Sometimes	Never
Disputing beliefs that support aggression	Always	Sometimes	Never
Catching one's own cognitive distortions	Always	Sometimes	Never

(cont.)

Checklist of Anger Management Skills *(page 2 of 2)*

Assertiveness and Social Skills:

Ignoring peer provocation	Always	Sometimes	Never
Escalating verbal assertion	Always	Sometimes	Never
Using "I" statements	Always	Sometimes	Never
Talking in a calm voice	Always	Sometimes	Never
Controlling nonverbal expressions	Always	Sometimes	Never
Modulating angry facial expressions	Always	Sometimes	Never
Making eye contact	Always	Sometimes	Never
Active listening	Always	Sometimes	Never
Apologizing when needed	Always	Sometimes	Never
Explaining one's own side of the story	Always	Sometimes	Never

Treatment Fidelity Checklist

General Instructions

Each CBT session consists of six to eight sections that correspond to the session's goals. The Treatment Fidelity Checklist rates the extent to which each of the session's goals has been accomplished. Some of the activities with each goal are repetitive and the therapists can use their clinical judgment to select those activities that are appropriate for the child. These decisions should be based on the child's age, motivation, and target symptoms. Goal attainment is rated on a 0 to 2 scale where:

0 = The child refused to engage in the activities of this goal or all activities for this goal were considered inappropriate or irrelevant for the child and not initiated by the therapist.

1 = The child was exposed to the rationale for the goal but did not fully engage in corresponding activities, such as discussions, role-plays, or working on handouts.

2 = The goal was attained and the therapeutic procedures were utilized in accordance with the child's age, motivation, and target symptoms.

By convention, treatment fidelity of 80% and above reflects adequate adherence to the manual.

Child's Behavior during the Session

The therapists can also rate the child's level of cooperation with in-session activities as well as the extent to which any behavioral, attentional, or affective problems that might have interfered with the session.

0 = no symptoms in this area were present.

1 = mild symptoms were present but didn't interfere with the session.

2 = symptoms were present and interfered with the session activities.

1. Poor compliance (low motivation, refusal) .... 0 .... 1 2
2. Hyperactive behaviors (fidgeting, getting out of seat) .... 0 .... 1 2
3. Inattention (difficulty focusing or maintaining attention) .... 0 .... 1 2
4. Mood (irritable, anxious, depressed) .... 0 .... 1 2

(cont.)

Treatment Fidelity Checklist for Session 1

Name or ID _____   Date _____/_____/_____

1. Present the rationale for treatment.	1	2	3
2. Review treatment goals.	1	2	3
3. Define anger and the elements of anger episodes.	1	2	3
4. Discuss the child's typical anger-provoking situations.	1	2	3
5. Discuss the frequency, intensity, and duration of recent anger episodes.	1	2	3
6. Discuss typical coping responses and introduce distraction and brief relaxation.	1	2	3
7. Summarize the session and assign homework.	1	2	3

Mean _____

Child's Behavior during the Session

1. Poor compliance (low motivation, refusal).	1	2	3
2. Hyperactive behaviors (fidgeting, getting out of seat).	1	2	3
3. Inattention (difficulty focusing or maintaining attention).	1	2	3
4. Mood (irritable, anxious, depressed).	1	2	3

Mean _____

Treatment Fidelity Checklist for Session 2

Name or ID _____ Date _____/_____/_____

1. Collect homework and review the last session's material.	1	2	3
2. Discuss anger intensity and the Feeling Thermometer technique.	1	2	3
3. Introduce the Stop & Think technique.	1	2	3
4. Discuss and practice using verbal reminders.	1	2	3
5. Discuss verbal labels for angry feelings.	1	2	3
6. Continue relaxation training.	1	2	3
7. Summarize the session and assign homework.	1	2	3

Mean _____

Child's Behavior during the Session

1. Poor compliance (low motivation, refusal).	1	2	3
2. Hyperactive behaviors (fidgeting, getting out of seat).	1	2	3
3. Inattention (difficulty focusing or maintaining attention).	1	2	3
4. Mood (irritable, anxious, depressed).	1	2	3

Mean _____

Treatment Fidelity Checklist for Session 3

Name or ID _____ Date _____/_____/_____

1. Collect homework and review the previous session's material.	1	2	3
2. Review progress to date.	1	2	3
3. Discuss ways to prevent anger-provoking situations.	1	2	3
4. Discuss the monitoring of anger cues.	1	2	3
5. Continue relaxation training: progressive muscle relaxation.	1	2	3
6. Summarize the session and assign homework.	1	2	3

Mean _____

Child's Behavior during the Session

1. Poor compliance (low motivation, refusal).	1	2	3
2. Hyperactive behaviors (fidgeting, getting out of seat).	1	2	3
3. Inattention (difficulty focusing or maintaining attention).	1	2	3
4. Mood (irritable, anxious, depressed).	1	2	3

Mean _____

Treatment Fidelity Checklist for Session 4

Name or ID _____ Date _____/_____/_____

1. Collect homework and review the previous session's material.   1   2   3

2. Discuss the connection between thoughts and emotions.   1   2   3

3. Introduce problem identification.   1   2   3

4. Discuss perspective taking.   1   2   3

5. Discuss hostile attribution bias.   1   2   3

6. Summarize the session and assign homework.   1   2   3

Mean _____

Child's Behavior during the Session

1. Poor compliance (low motivation, refusal).   1   2   3

2. Hyperactive behaviors (fidgeting, getting out of seat).   1   2   3

3. Inattention (difficulty focusing or maintaining attention).   1   2   3

4. Mood (irritable, anxious, depressed).   1   2   3

Mean _____

Treatment Fidelity Checklist for Session 5

Name or ID _____ Date _____/_____/_____

1. Collect homework and review the previous session's material.	1	2	3
2. Introduce the PICC handout.	1	2	3
3. Practice generating a range of solutions to problem situations.	1	2	3
4. Discuss the effects of anger on problem-solving ability.	1	2	3
5. Reinforce the use of appropriate verbal solutions.	1	2	3
6. Summarize the session and assign homework.	1	2	3

Mean _____

Child's Behavior during the Session

1. Poor compliance (low motivation, refusal).	1	2	3
2. Hyperactive behaviors (fidgeting, getting out of seat).	1	2	3
3. Inattention (difficulty focusing or maintaining attention).	1	2	3
4. Mood (irritable, anxious, depressed).	1	2	3

Mean _____

Treatment Fidelity Checklist for Session 6

Name or ID _____ Date _____/_____/_____

	1	2	3
1. Collect homework and review the previous session's material.	1	2	3
2. Introduce consequential thinking.	1	2	3
3. Discuss consequences for other people.	1	2	3
4. Practice consequential thinking.	1	2	3
5. Troubleshoot resistance to problem-solving training.	1	2	3
6. Summarize the session and assign homework.	1	2	3

Mean _____

Child's Behavior during the Session

	1	2	3
1. Poor compliance (low motivation, refusal).	1	2	3
2. Hyperactive behaviors (fidgeting, getting out of seat).	1	2	3
3. Inattention (difficulty focusing or maintaining attention).	1	2	3
4. Mood (irritable, anxious, depressed).	1	2	3

Mean _____

Treatment Fidelity Checklist for Session 7

Name or ID _____ Date _____ / _____ / _____

1. Collect homework and review the previous session's material.		1	2	3
2. Introduce social skills training.		1	2	3
3. Define and discuss assertive behavior and de-escalation.		1	2	3
4. Develop a coping template for peer provocation.		1	2	3
5. Practice assertiveness skills.		1	2	3
6. Discuss nonverbal aspects of social interaction.		1	2	3
7. Summarize the session and assign homework.		1	2	3

Mean _____

Child's Behavior during the Session

1. Poor compliance (low motivation, refusal).		1	2	3
2. Hyperactive behaviors (fidgeting, getting out of seat).		1	2	3
3. Inattention (difficulty focusing or maintaining attention).		1	2	3
4. Mood (irritable, anxious, depressed).		1	2	3

Mean _____

Treatment Fidelity Checklist for Session 8

Name or ID _____ Date _____/_____/_____

1. Collect homework and review the previous session's material.	1	2	3
2. Discuss fairness and rights.	1	2	3
3. Role-play social skills when rights have been violated.	1	2	3
4. Practice active listening skills.	1	2	3
5. Develop a coping template for dealing with accusation.	1	2	3
6. Summarize the session and assign homework.	1	2	3

Mean _____

Child's Behavior during the Session

1. Poor compliance (low motivation, refusal).	1	2	3
2. Hyperactive behaviors (fidgeting, getting out of seat).	1	2	3
3. Inattention (difficulty focusing or maintaining attention).	1	2	3
4. Mood (irritable, anxious, depressed).	1	2	3

Mean _____

Treatment Fidelity Checklist for Session 9

Name or ID _____ Date _____/_____/_____

1. Collect homework and review the previous session's material.	1	2	3
2. Develop a coping template for conflicts with adults.	1	2	3
3. Discuss situations that lead to conflicts at home.	1	2	3
4. Practice monitoring poor communication habits.	1	2	3
5. Practice explaining one's role in a conflict situation.	1	2	3
6. Summarize the session and assign homework.	1	2	3

Mean _____

Child's Behavior during the Session

1. Poor compliance (low motivation, refusal).	1	2	3
2. Hyperactive behaviors (fidgeting, getting out of seat).	1	2	3
3. Inattention (difficulty focusing or maintaining attention).	1	2	3
4. Mood (irritable, anxious, depressed).	1	2	3

Mean _____

Treatment Fidelity Checklist for Session 10

Name or ID _____ Date _____ / _____ / _____

1. Collect homework and review the previous session's material.	1	2	3
2. Obtain the child's feedback on program effectiveness.	1	2	3
3. Conduct additional program review procedures.	1	2	3
4. Present the graduation diploma.	1	2	3

Mean _____

Child's Behavior during the Session

1. Poor compliance (low motivation, refusal).	1	2	3
2. Hyperactive behaviors (fidgeting, getting out of seat).	1	2	3
3. Inattention (difficulty focusing or maintaining attention).	1	2	3
4. Mood (irritable, anxious, depressed).	1	2	3

Mean _____

References

Achenbach, T. M. (1991). *Manual for the Child Behavior Checklist/4–18 and 1991 profile.* Burlington: University of Vermont Press.

Achenbach, T. M., Conners, C. K., Quay, H. C., Verhulst, F. C., & Howell, C. T. (1989). Replication of empirically derived syndromes as a basis for taxonomy of child/adolescent psychopathology. *Journal of Abnormal Child Psychology, 17*(3), 299–323.

Aman, M. G., McDougle, C. J., Scahill, L., Handen, B., Arnold, L. E., Johnson, C., et al. (2009). Medication and parent training in children with pervasive developmental disorders and serious behavior problems: Results from a randomized clinical trial. *Journal of the American Academy of Child and Adolescent Psychiatry, 48*(12), 1143–1154.

Aman, M. G., Singh, N. N., Stewart, A. W., & Field, C. J. (1985). The Aberrant Behavior Checklist: A behavior rating scale for the assessment of treatment effects. *American Journal of Mental Deficiency, 89*(5), 485–491.

American Psychiatric Association. (2000). *Diagnostic and statistical manual of mental disorders* (4th ed., text rev.). Washington, DC: Author.

Armbruster, P., Sukhodolsky, D., & Michalsen, R. (2004). The impact of managed care on children's outpatient treatment: A comparison study of treatment outcome before and after managed care. *American Journal of Orthopsychiatry, 74*(1), 5–13.

Armenteros, J. L., & Lewis, J. E. (2002). Citalopram treatment for impulsive aggression in children and adolescents: An open pilot study. *Journal of the American Academy of Child and Adolescent Psychiatry, 41*(5), 522–529.

Arnold, L. E., Vitiello, B., McDougle, C., Scahill, L., Shah, B., Gonzalez, N. M., et al. (2003). Parent-defined target symptoms respond to risperidone in RUPP Autism Study: Customer approach to clinical trials. *Journal of the American Academy of Child and Adolescent Psychiatry, 42*(12), 1443–1450.

Ash, P., & Nurcombe, B. (2007). Malpractice and professional liability. In A. Martin & F. Volkmar (Eds.), *Lewis's child and adolescent psychiatry* (pp. 1018–1031). Philadelphia: Lippincott Williams & Wilkins.

Averill, J. R. (1983). Studies on anger and aggression: Implications for theories of emotion. *American Psychologist, 38*(11), 1145–1160.

Bandura, A. (1973). *Aggression: A social learning analysis.* Oxford, UK: Prentice-Hall.

Barkley, R. A. (1997). *Defiant children: A clinician's manual for assessment and parent training* (2nd ed.). New York: Guilford Press.

Barkley, R. A., Edwards, G., Laneri, M., Fletcher, K., & Metevia, L. (2001). The efficacy of problem-solving communication training alone, behavior management training alone, and their combination for parent–adolescent conflict in teenagers with ADHD and ODD. *Journal of Consulting and Clinical Psychology, 69*(6), 926–941.

Barkley, R. A., Edwards, G. H., & Robin, A. L. (1999). *Defiant teens: A clinician's manual for assessment and family intervention.* New York: Guilford Press.

Barratt, E. S., Kent, T. A., Felthous, A., & Stanford, M. S. (1997). Neuropsychological and cognitive psychophysiological substrates of impulsive aggression. *Biological Psychiatry, 41*(10), 1045–1061.

Benson, B. A., & Aman, M. G. (1999). Disruptive behavior disorders in children with mental retardation. In H. C. Quay & A. E. Hogan (Eds.), *Handbook of disruptive behavior disorders* (pp. 559–578). Dordrecht, The Netherlands: Kluwer Academic.

Berkowitz, L. (1990). On the formation and regulation of anger and aggression: A cognitive-neoassociationistic analysis. *American Psychologist, 45*(4), 494–503.

Blanchard-Fields, F., & Coats, A. H. (2008). The experience of anger and sadness in everyday problems impacts age differences in emotion regulation. *Developmental Psychology, 44*(6), 1547–1556.

Borduin, C. M., Mann, B. J., Cone, L. T., Henggeler, S. W., Fucci, B. R., Blaske, D. M., et al. (1995). Multisystemic treatment of serious juvenile offenders: Long-term prevention of criminality and violence. *Journal of Consulting and Clinical Psychology, 63*(4), 569–578.

Borum, R. (2000). Assessing violence risk among youth. *Journal of Clinical Psychology, 56*(10), 1263–1288.

Borum, R., Fein, R., Vossekuil, B., & Berglund, J. (1999). Threat assessment: Defining an approach for evaluating risk of targeted violence. *Behavioral Sciences and the Law, 17*(3), 323–337.

Bourke, M. L., & Van Hasselt, V. B. (2001). Social problem-solving skills training for incarcerated offenders: A treatment manual. *Behavior Modification, 25*(2), 163–188.

Bronfenbrenner, U. (1979). Contexts of child rearing: Problems and prospects. *American Psychologist, 34*(10), 844–850.

Brown, E. C., Aman, M. G., & Havercamp, S. M. (2002). Factor analysis and norms for parent ratings on the Aberrant Behavior Checklist—Community for young people in special education. *Research in Developmental Disabilities, 23*(1), 45–60.

Brunner, T. M., & Spielberger, C. D. (2009). *State–Trait Anger Expression Inventory–2: Child and Adolescent.* Lutz, FL: Psychological Assessment Resources.

Bubier, J. L., & Drabick, D. A. G. (2009). Co-occurring anxiety and disruptive behavior disorders: The roles of anxious symptoms, reactive aggression, and shared risk processes. *Clinical Psychology Review, 29*(7), 658–669.

Carlson, G. A. (2007). Who are the children with severe mood dysregulation, a.k.a. "rages"? *American Journal of Psychiatry, 164*(8), 1140–1142.

Collett, B. R., Ohan, J. L., & Myers, K. M. (2003). Ten-year review of rating scales: VI. Scales assessing externalizing behaviors. *Journal of the American Academy of Child and Adolescent Psychiatry, 42*(10), 1143–1170.

Costello, E. J., Mustillo, S., Erkanli, A., Keeler, G., & Angold, A. (2003). Prevalence and development of psychiatric disorders in childhood and adolescence. *Archives of General Psychiatry, 60*(8), 837–844.

Crick, N. R., & Dodge, K. A. (1994). A review and reformulation of social information-processing mechanisms in children's social adjustment. *Psychological Bulletin, 115*(1), 74–101.

Deater-Deckard, K. (2001). Annotation: Recent research examining the role of peer relationships in the development of psychopathology. *Journal of Child Psychology and Psychiatry and Allied Disciplines, 42*(5), 565–579.

Deffenbacher, J. L., Lynch, R. S., Oetting, E. R., & Kemper, C. C. (1996). Anger reduction in early adolescents. *Journal of Counseling Psychology, 43*(2), 149–157.

DiGuiseppe, R., & Tafrate, R. C. (2003). Anger treatment for adults: A meta-analytic review. *Clinical Psychology: Science and Practice, 10*(1), 70–84.

Dodge, K. A. (1980). Social cognition and children's aggressive behavior. *Child Development, 51*(1), 162–170.

Dodge, K. A. (2003). Do social information-processing patterns mediate aggressive behavior? In B. B. Lahey, T. E. Moffitt, & A. Caspi (Eds.), *Causes of conduct disorder and juvenile delinquency* (pp. 254–274). New York: Guilford Press.

Dodge, K. A. (2006). Translational science in action: Hostile attributional style and the development of aggressive behavior problems. *Development and Psychopathology, 18*(3), 791–814.

Dodge, K. A., Bates, J. E., & Pettit, G. S. (1990). Mechanisms in the cycle of violence. *Science, 250,* 1678–1683.

Dollard, J., Dood, L., Miller, N., Mowrer, O., & Sears, R. (1939). *Frustration and aggression.* New Haven, CT: Yale University Press.

Donovan, S. J., Stewart, J. W., Nunes, E. V., Quitkin, F. M., Parides, M., Daniel, W., et al. (2000). Divalproex treatment for youth with explosive temper and mood lability: A double-blind, placebo-controlled crossover design. *American Journal of Psychiatry, 157*(5), 818–820.

DuPaul, G. J., & Barkley, R. A. (1992). Situational variability of attention problems: Psychometric properties of the Revised Home and School Situations Questionnaires. *Journal of Clinical Child Psychology, 21*(2), 178–188.

D'Zurilla, T. J., & Goldfried, M. R. (1971). Problem solving and behavior modification. *Journal of Abnormal Psychology, 78*(1), 107–126.

Eaton, D. K., Kann, L., Kinchen, S., Ross, J., Hawkins, J., Harris, W. A., et al. (2006). Youth risk behavior surveillance—United States, 2005. *Morbidity and Mortality Weekly Report, Surveillance Summaries/CDC, 55*(5), 1–108.

Eckhardt, C., Norlander, B., & Deffenbacher, J. (2004). The assessment of anger and hostility: A critical review. *Aggression and Violent Behavior,* 9(1), 17–43.

Ekman, P. (1993). Facial expression and emotion. *American Psychologist, 48*(4), 384–392.

Ellis, A. (2002). *Anger: How to live with and without it.* New York: Citadel Press.

Feindler, E. L., & Ecton, R. B. (1986). *Adolescent anger control: Cognitive-behavioral techniques.* New York: Pergamon Press.

Feindler, E. L., Ecton, R. B., Kingsley, D., & Dubey, D. R. (1986). Group anger-control training for institutionalized psychiatric male adolescents. *Behavior Therapy, 17*(2), 109–123.

Feindler, E. L., Marriott, S. A., & Iwata, M. (1984). Group anger control training for junior high school delinquents. *Cognitive Therapy and Research, 8*(3), 299–311.

Fergusson, D. M., & Horwood, L. J. (2002). Male and female offending trajectories. *Development and Psychopathology, 14*(1), 159–177.

Frick, P. J., Lahey, B. B., Loeber, R., Tannenbaum, L., Van Horn, Y., Christ, M. A. G., et al. (1993). Oppositional defiant disorder and conduct disorder: A meta-analytic review of factor analyses and cross-validation in a clinic sample. *Clinical Psychology Review, 13*(4), 319–340.

Garrison, S. R., & Stolberg, A. L. (1983). Modification of anger in children by affective imagery training. *Journal of Abnormal Child Psychology, 11*(1), 115–129.

Gershoff, E. T. (2002). Corporal punishment by parents and associated child behaviors and experiences: A meta-analytic and theoretical review. *Psychological Bulletin, 128*(4), 539–579.

Goldbeck, L., & Schmid, K. (2003). Effectiveness of autogenic relaxation training on children and adolescents with behavioral and emotional problems. *Journal of the American Academy of Child and Adolescent Psychiatry, 42*(9), 1046–1054.

Goldstein, A. P., & Glick, B. (1987). *Aggression replacement training: A comprehensive intervention for aggressive youth.* Champaign, IL: Research Press.

Gomez, R., Burns, G. L., & Walsh, J. A. (2008). Parent ratings of the oppositional defiant disorder symptoms: Item response theory analyses of cross-national and cross-racial invariance. *Journal of Psychopathology and Behavioral Assessment, 30*, 10–19.

Grodnitzky, G. R., & Tafrate, R. C. (2000). Imaginal exposure for anger reduction in adult outpatients: A pilot study. *Journal of Behavior Therapy and Experimental Psychiatry, 31*(3–4), 259–279.

Guerra, N. G., & Slaby, R. G. (1990). Cognitive mediators of aggression in adolescent offenders: 2. Intervention. *Developmental Psychology, 26*(2), 269–277.

Hazaleus, S. L., & Deffenbacher, J. L. (1986). Relaxation and cognitive treatments of anger. *Journal of Consulting and Clinical Psychology, 54*(2), 222–226.

Henggeler, S. W., Brondino, M. J., Melton, G. B., Scherer, D. G., & Hanley, J. H. (1997). Multisystemic therapy with violent and chronic juvenile offenders and their families: The role of treatment fidelity in successful dissemination. *Journal of Consulting and Clinical Psychology, 65*(5), 821–833.

Henggeler, S. W., Melton, G. B., & Smith, L. A. (1992). Family preservation using multisystemic therapy: An effective alternative to incarcerating serious juvenile offenders. *Journal of Consulting and Clinical Psychology, 60*(6), 953–961.

Henggeler, S. W., Pickrel, S. G., & Brondino, M. J. (1999). Multisystemic treatment of substance-abusing and dependent delinquents: Outcomes, treatment fidelity, and transportability. *Mental Health Services Research, 1*(3), 171–184.

Henggeler, S. W., Rowland, M. D., Randall, J., Pickrel, S. G., Cunningham, P. B., Miller, S. L., et al. (1999). Home-based multisystemic therapy as an alternative to the hospitalization of youths in psychiatric crisis: Clinical outcomes. *Journal of the American Academy of Child and Adolescent Psychiatry, 38*(11), 1331–1339.

Hudley, C., & Graham, S. (1993). An attributional intervention to reduce peer-directed aggression among African-American boys. *Child Development, 64*(1), 124–138.

Jarvis, P. (2006). "Rough and tumble" play: Lessons in life. *Evolutionary Psychology, 4*, 330–346.

Jensen, P. S., Pappadopulos, E., Schur, S. B., Siennick, S. E., Jensen, P. S., MacIntyre, J. C. II, et al. (2003). Treatment recommendations for the use of antipsychotics for aggressive youth (TRAAY): Part II. *Journal of the American Academy of Child and Adolescent Psychiatry, 42*(2), 145–161.

Kassinove, H., & Sukhodolsky, D. G. (1995). Anger disorders: Basic science and practice issues. *Issues in Comprehensive Pediatric Nursing, 18*(3), 173–205.

Kassinove, H., Sukhodolsky, D. G., Tsytsarev, S. V., & Solovyova, S. (1997). Self-reported anger episodes in Russia and America. *Journal of Social Behavior and Personality, 12*(2), 301–324.

Kassinove, H., & Tafrate, R. C. (2002). *Anger management: The complete treatment guidebook for practitioners.* Atascadero, CA: Impact Publishers.

Kaufman, J., Birmaher, B., Brent, D., Rao, U., Flynn, C., Moreci, P., et al. (1997). Schedule for Affective Disorders and Schizophrenia for School-Age Children—Present and Lifetime Version (K-SADS-PL): Initial reliability and validity data. *Journal of the American Academy of Child and Adolescent Psychiatry, 36*(7), 980–988.

Kazdin, A. E. (2005). *Parent management training: Treatment for oppositional, aggressive, and antisocial behavior in children and adolescents.* New York: Oxford University Press.

Kazdin, A. E., Esveldt-Dawson, K., French, N. H., & Unis, A. S. (1987). Problem-solving skills training and relationship therapy in the treatment of antisocial child behavior. *Journal of Consulting and Clinical Psychology, 55*(1), 76–85.

Kazdin, A. E., Siegel, T. C., & Bass, D. (1992). Cognitive problem-solving skills training and parent management training in the treatment of antisocial behavior in children. *Journal of Consulting and Clinical Psychology, 60*(5), 733–747.

Keenan, K., & Wakschlag, L. S. (2004). Are oppositional defiant and conduct disorder symptoms normative behaviors in preschoolers?: A comparison of referred and nonreferred children. *American Journal of Psychiatry, 161*(2), 356–358.

Kellner, M. H. (2001). *In control: A skill-building program for teaching young adolescents to manage anger.* Champain, IL: Research Press.

Kendall, P. C. (2006). Guiding theory for therapy with children and adolescents. In P. C. Kendall (Ed.), *Child and adolescent therapy: Cognitive-behavioral procedures* (3rd ed., pp. 3–30). New York: Guilford Press.

Kendall, P. C., Chu, B., Gifford, A., Hayes, C., & Nauta, M. (1998). Breathing life into a manual: Flexibility and creativity with manual-based treatments. *Cognitive and Behavioral Practice, 5*(2), 177–198.

Kjelsberg, E. (2002). Pathways to violent and nonviolent criminality in an adolescent psychiatric population. *Child Psychiatry and Human Development, 33*(1), 29–42.

Kolko, D. J., Herschell, A. D., & Scharf, D. M. (2006). Education and treatment for boys who set fires: Specificity, moderators, and predictors of recidivism. *Journal of Emotional and Behavioral Disorders, 14*(4), 227–239.

Kraemer, H. C., Measelle, J. R., Ablow, J. C., Essex, M. J., Boyce, W. T., & Kupfer, D. J. (2003). A new approach to integrating data from multiple informants in psychiatric assessment and research: Mixing and matching contexts and perspectives. *American Journal of Psychiatry, 160*(9), 1566–1577.

Kraijer, D. (2000). Review of adaptive behavior studies in mentally retarded persons with autism/pervasive developmental disorder. *Journal of Autism and Developmental Disorders, 30*(1), 39–47.

Lahey, B. B., Loeber, R., Quay, H. C., Applegate, B., Shaffer, D., Waldman, I., et al. (1998). Validity of DSM-IV subtypes of conduct disorder based on age of onset. *Journal of the American Academy of Child and Adolescent Psychiatry, 37*(4), 435–442.

Leibenluft, E., Blair, R. J., Charney, D. S., & Pine, D. S. (2003). Irritability in pediatric mania and other childhood psychopathology. *Annals of the New York Academy of Sciences, 1008,* 201–218.

Leve, L. D., Chamberlain, P., & Reid, J. B. (2005). Intervention outcomes for girls referred from juvenile justice: Effects on delinquency. *Journal of Consulting and Clinical Psychology, 73*(6), 1181–1184.

Lipsey, M. W., & Wilson, D. B. (1998). Effective intervention for serious juvenile offenders: A synthesis of research. In R. Loeber & D. P. Farrington (Eds.), *Serious and violent juvenile offenders: Risk factors and successful interventions* (pp. 86–105). Thousand Oaks, CA: Sage.

Lochman, J. E., Barry, T. D., & Pardini, D. A. (2003). Anger control training for aggressive youth. In A. E. Kazdin & J. R. Weisz (Eds.), *Evidence-based psychotherapies for children and adolescents* (pp. 263–281). New York: Guilford Press.

Lochman, J. E., Curry, J. F., Burch, P. R., & Lampron, L. B. (1984). Treatment and generalization effects of cognitive-behavioral and goal-setting interventions with aggressive boys. *Journal of Consulting and Clinical Psychology, 52*(5), 915–916.

Lochman, J. E., & Wells, K. C. (2004). The Coping Power Program for preadolescent aggressive boys and their parents: Outcome effects at the 1-year follow-up. *Journal of Consulting and Clinical Psychology, 72*(4), 571–578.

Lochman, J. E., Wells, K. C., & Lenhart, L. A. (2008). *Coping Power: Child group program.* New York: Oxford University Press.

Lochman, J. E., Whidby, J. M., & FizGerald, D. P. (2000). Cognitive-behavioral assessment and treatment with aggressive children. In P. C. Kendall (Ed.), *Child and adolescent therapy: Cognitive-behavioral procedures* (2nd ed., pp. 31–87). New York: Guilford Press.

Loeber, R., Green, S. M., Kalb, L., Lahey, B. B., & Loeber, R. (2000). Physical fighting in childhood as a risk factor for later mental health problems. *Journal of the American Academy of Child and Adolescent Psychiatry, 39*(4), 421–428.

Losel, F., & Beelmann, A. (2003). Effects of child skills training in preventing antisocial behavior: A systematic review of randomized evaluations. *Annals of the American Academy of Political and Social Science, 587,* 84–109.

Luborsky, L., & DeRubeis, R. J. (1984). The use of psychotherapy treatment manuals: A small revolution in psychotherapy research style. *Clinical Psychology Review, 4,* 5–14.

Malone, R. P., Delaney, M. A., Luebbert, J. F.,

Cater, J., & Campbell, M. (2000). A double-blind placebo-controlled study of lithium in hospitalized aggressive children and adolescents with conduct disorder. *Archives of General Psychiatry, 57*(7), 649–654.

Maughan, B., Rowe, R., Pickles, A., Costello, E. J., & Angold, A. (2000). Developmental trajectories of aggressive and non-aggressive conduct problems. *Journal of Quantitative Criminology, 16*(2), 199–221.

McMahon, R. J., & Forehand, R. L. (2003). *Helping the noncompliant child: Family-based treatment for oppositional behavior* (2nd ed.). New York: Guilford Press.

Meichenbaum, D., & Cameron, R. (1973). *Stress inoculation: A skills training approach to anxiety management.* Waterloo, Ontario, Canada: University of Waterloo.

Merrell, K. W., & Gimpel, G. A. (1998). *Social skills of children and adolescents: Conceptualization, assessment, treatment.* Mahwah, NJ: Erlbaum.

Minuchin, S. (1974). *Families and family therapy.* Cambridge, MA: Harvard University Press.

MTA Cooperative Group. (1999). A 14-month randomized clinical trial of treatment strategies for attention-deficit/hyperactivity disorder: The MTA Cooperative Group Multimodal Treatment Study of Children with ADHD. *Archives of General Psychiatry, 56*(12), 1073–1086.

Nagin, D., & Tremblay, R. E. (1999). Trajectories of boys' physical aggression, opposition, and hyperactivity on the path to physically violent and nonviolent juvenile delinquency. *Child Development, 70*(5), 1181–1196.

Nelson, W. M., & Finch, A. J. (2000). *Children's Inventory of Anger.* Los Angeles: Western Psychological Services.

Novaco, R. W. (1975). *Anger control: The development and evaluation of experimental treatment.* Lexington, MA: Health.

Office of Juvenile Justice and Delinquency Prevention. (2008). *Girls Study Group: Understanding and responding to girls' delinquency.* Washington, DC: U.S. Department of Justice, Office of Justice Programs.

Patterson, G. R., DeBaryshe, B. D., & Ramsey, E. (1989). A developmental perspective on antisocial behavior. *American Psychologist, 44*(2), 329–335.

Patterson, G. R., Reid, J. B., & Dishion, T. J. (1992). *A social learning approach: IV. Antisocial boys.* Eugene, OR: Castalia.

Pavuluri, M. N., Birmaher, B., & Naylor, M. W. (2005). Pediatric bipolar disorder: A review of the past 10 years. *Journal of the American Academy of Child and Adolescent Psychiatry, 44*(9), 846–871.

Perepletchikova, F., & Kazdin, A. E. (2005). Treatment integrity and therapeutic change: Issues and research recommendations. *Clinical Psychology: Science and Practice, 12*(4), 365–383.

Potegal, M., & Davidson, R. J. (2003). Temper tantrums in young children: 1. Behavioral composition. *Journal of Developmental and Behavioral Pediatrics, 24*(3), 140–147.

Potegal, M., Kosorok, M. R., & Davidson, R. J. (2003). Temper tantrums in young children: 2. Tantrum duration and temporal organization. *Journal of Developmental and Behavioral Pediatrics, 24*(3), 148–154.

Rice, B. J., Woolston, J., Stewart, E., Kerker, B. D., & Horwitz, S. M. (2002). Differences in younger, middle, and older children admitted to child psychiatric inpatient services. *Child Psychiatry and Human Development, 32*(4), 241–261.

RUPP Autism Network. (2002). Risperidone in children with autism and serious behavioral problems. *New England Journal of Medicine, 347*(5), 314–321.

Scahill, L., Sukhodolsky, D. G., Bearss, K., Findley, D. B., Hamrin, V., Carroll, D. H., et al. (2006). A randomized trial of parent management training in children with tic disorders and disruptive behavior. *Journal of Child Neurology, 21*(8), 650–656.

Schaeffer, C. M., & Borduin, C. M. (2005). Long-term follow-up to a randomized clinical trial of multisystemic therapy with serious and violent juvenile offenders. *Journal of Consulting and Clinical Psychology, 73*(3), 445–453.

Schur, S. B., Sikich, L., Findling, R. L., Malone, R. P., Crismon, M. L., Derivan, A., et al. (2003). Treatment recommendations for the use of antipsychotics for aggressive youth (TRAAY): Part I. A review. *Journal of the American Academy of Child and Adolescent Psychiatry, 42*(2), 132–144.

Shure, M. B. (1993). I can problem solve (ICPS): Interpersonal cognitive problem solving for young children. *Early Child Development and Care, 96*, 49–64.

Shure, M. B., & Spivack, G. (1972). Means–ends thinking, adjustment, and social class among elementary-school-aged children. *Journal of Consulting and Clinical Psychology, 38*(3), 348–353.

Shure, M. B., & Spivack, G. (1982). Interpersonal problem-solving in young children: A cognitive approach to prevention. *American Journal of Community Psychology, 10*(3), 341–356.

Silver, J. M., & Yudofsky, S. C. (1991). The Overt Aggression Scale: Overview and guiding principles. *Journal of Neuropsychiatry and Clinical Neurosciences, 3*(2), S22–S29.

Silverthorn, P., & Frick, P. J. (1999). Developmental pathways to antisocial behavior: The delayed-onset pathway in girls. *Development and Psychopathology*, *11*(1), 101–126.

Skinner, B. F. (1938). *The behavior of organisms: An experimental analysis*. New York: Free Press.

Snyder, K. V., Kymissis, P., Kessler, K., & Snyder, K. V. (1999). Anger management for adolescents: Efficacy of brief group therapy. *Journal of the American Academy of Child and Adolescent Psychiatry*, *38*(11), 1409–1416.

Spence, S. H. (2003). Social skills training with children and young people: Theory, evidence and practice. *Child and Adolescent Mental Health*, *8*(2), 84–96.

Spielberger, C. D. (1988). *Manual for the State–Trait Anger Expression Inventory (STAXI)*. Odessa, FL: Psychological Assessment Resources.

Sukhodolsky, D. G., & Butter, E. (2006). Social skills training for children with intellectual disabilities. In J. W. Jacobson & J. A. Mulick (Eds.), *Handbook of mental retardation and developmental disabilities* (pp. 601–618). New York: Kluwer.

Sukhodolsky, D. G., Cardona, L., & Martin, A. (2005). Characterizing aggressive and noncompliant behaviors in a children's psychiatric inpatient setting. *Child Psychiatry and Human Development*, *36*(2), 177–193.

Sukhodolsky, D. G., Golub, A., & Cromwell, E. N. (2001). Development and validation of the Anger Rumination Scale. *Personality and Individual Differences*, *31*(5), 689–700.

Sukhodolsky, D. G., Golub, A., Stone, E. C., & Orban, L. (2005). Dismantling anger control training for children: A randomized pilot study of social problem-solving versus social skills training components. *Behavior Therapy*, *36*(1), 15–23.

Sukhodolsky, D. G., Kassinove, H., & Gorman, B. S. (2004). Cognitive-behavioral therapy for anger in children and adolescents: A meta-analysis. *Aggression and Violent Behavior*, *9*(3), 247–269.

Sukhodolsky, D. G., & Ruchkin, V. (2006). Evidence-based psychosocial treatments in the juvenile justice system. *Child and Adolescent Psychiatric Clinics of North America*, *15*(2), 501–516.

Sukhodolsky, D. G., & Ruchkin, V. V. (2004). Association of normative beliefs and anger with aggression and antisocial behavior in Russian male juvenile offenders and high school students. *Journal of Abnormal Child Psychology*, *32*(2), 225–236.

Sukhodolsky, D. G., Solomon, R. M., & Perine, J. (2000). Cognitive-behavioral, anger-control intervention for elementary school children: A treatment outcome study. *Journal of Child and Adolescent Group Therapy*, *10*(3), 159–170.

Sukhodolsky, D. G., Vitulano, L. A., Carroll, D. H., McGuire, J., Leckman, J. F., & Scahill, L. (2009). Randomized trial of anger control training for adolescents with Tourette's Syndrome and disruptive behavior. *Journal of the American Academy of Child and Adolescent Psychiatry*, *48*(4), 413–421.

Suls, J., & Bunde, J. (2005). Anger, anxiety, and depression as risk factors for cardiovascular disease: The problems and implications of overlapping affective dispositions. *Psychological Bulletin*, *131*(2), 260–300.

Swearer, S. M., Espelage, D. L., & Napolitano, S. A. (2009). *Bullying prevention and intervention: Realistic strategies for schools*. New York: Guilford Press.

Tafrate, R. C., & Kassinove, H. (1998). Anger control in men: Barb exposure with rational, irrational, and irrelevant self-statements. *Journal of Cognitive Psychotherapy: An International Quarterly*, *12*(3), 187–211.

Vitiello, B., & Stoff, D. M. (1997). Subtypes of aggression and their relevance to child psychiatry. *Journal of the American Academy of Child and Adolescent Psychiatry*, *36*(3), 307–315.

Wakschlag, L. S., Tolan, P. H., & Leventhal, B. L. (2010). Research review: "Ain't misbehavin'": Towards a developmentally-specified nosology for preschool disruptive behavior. *Journal of Child Psychology and Psychiatry and Allied Disciplines*, *51*(1), 1–22.

Webster-Stratton, C., Hollinsworth, T., & Kolpacoff, M. (1989). The long-term effectiveness and clinical significance of three cost-effective training programs for families with conduct-problem children. *Journal of Consulting and Clinical Psychology*, *57*(4), 550–553.

Weisbrot, D. M., & Ettinger, A. B. (2002). Aggression and violence in mood disorders. *Child and Adolescent Psychiatric Clinics of North America*, *11*(3), 649–671.

Weisz, J. R., & Weiss, B. (1993). *Effects of psychotherapy with children and adolescents*. Thousand Oaks, CA: Sage.

Wolpe, J. (1958). *Psychotherapy by reciprocal inhibition*. Stanford, CA: Stanford University Press.

Wozniak, J., Biederman, J., Kiely, K., Ablon, J. S., Faraone, S. V., Mundy, E., et al. (1995). Mania-like symptoms suggestive of childhood-onset bipolar disorder in clinically referred children. *Journal of the American Academy of Child and Adolescent Psychiatry*, *34*(7), 867–876.

Yudofsky, S. C., Silver, J. M., Jackson, W., Endicott, J., & Williams, D. (1986). The Overt Aggression Scale for the objective rating of verbal and physical aggression. *American Journal of Psychiatry*, *143*(1), 35–39.

Index